MW00677061

ALKALINE DIET COOKBOOK
MADE EASY: 2 BOOKS IN 1

50+ Mouth-Watering, Simple, and Very Simple Recipes tp Cleanse you Body, Lose Fat, and Get Healthy in this Bundle of 2 Books About Alkaline Diet Cookbook Made Easy.

BY

Angela Bond

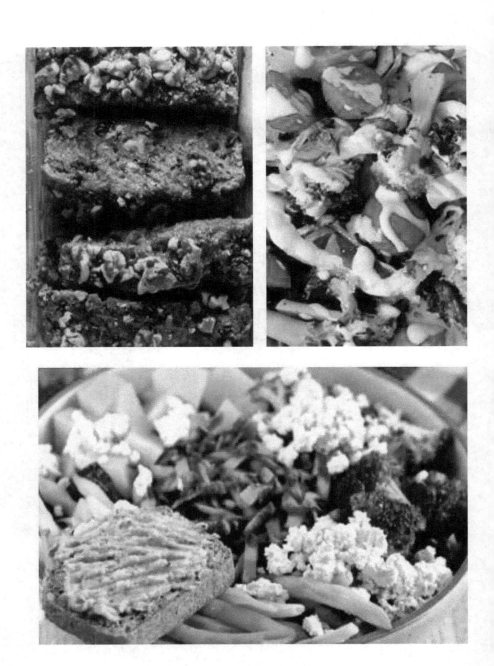

Copyrights Content Page

The content contained within this book may not be reproduced, duplicated or transmitted without direct written permission from the author or the publisher. Under no circumstances will any blame or legal responsibility be held against the publisher, or author, for any damages, reparation, or monetary loss due to the information contained within this book. Either directly or indirectly.

Legal Notice:

This book is copyright protected. This book is only for personal use. You cannot amend, distribute, sell, use, quote or paraphrase any part, or the content within this book, without the consent of the author or publisher.

Disclaimer Notice:

Please note the information contained within this document is for educational and entertainment purposes only. All effort has been executed to present accurate, up to date, and reliable, complete information. No warranties of any kind are declared or implied. Readers acknowledge that the author is not engaging in the rendering of legal, financial, medical or professional advice. The content within this book has been derived from various sources.

Please consult a licensed professional before attempting any techniques outlined in this book. By reading this document, the reader agrees that under no circumstances is the author responsible for any losses, direct or indirect, which are incurred as a result of the use of information contained within this document, including, but not limited to, errors, omissions, or inaccuracies.

ALKALINE DIET COOKBOOK MADE EASY FOR BEGINNERS

ALKALINE COOKBOOK MADE EASY FOR BEGINNERS

ALKALINE DIET COOKBOOK
MADE EASY FOR BEGINNERS

Table of Contents

Table of Contents

INTRODUCTION

The primary factor in the alkaline diet is balance. In sound individuals, a diet of 65% (by weight) alkaline-outlining food assortments and 35% destructive molding capacities commendably. For example, in the event that you by one way or another figured out how to have a 8-ounce steak for dinner, you'd need to eat around 23 ounces of alkaline-forming food sources during the day to keep up the 65-35 extent. In those with prosperity challenges, a 80-20 extent of alkaline-forming to destructive outlining food assortments is proposed, essentially because it reduces the proportion of effort your body needs to put into decreasing its destructive weight. (This implies 40 ounces of alkaline-forming food assortments as compensation for your 8-ounce steak — or you could essentially downsize your steak to 4 ounces taking everything into account.).

Regardless of the way that blood pH ought to stay stable in a slim extent of 7.35–7.45 for perseverance, the same isn't substantial for the pH of various fluids like pee and salivation, as these will move for the length of the day. The pH of the pee goes all over as demonstrated by the food sources we eat, exercise, stress, and various elements. The kidney is the fundamental organ responsible for buffering and releasing metabolic acids, anyway the kidney can't release pee that is more acidic than a pH of 4.5, as pee this destructive would duplicate the touchy tissues of the kidney. Oddly, if you eat an uncommonly destructive outlining dinner, your pee will routinely show an alkaline several hours afterward. You may think this implies that incredible essential pH balance; regardless, this is the effect of the pancreas making high proportions of alkalizing stomach related combinations as a result of the destructive molding food assortments ingested.

Alkaline diet meals

1.   Vegan Poke Bowl

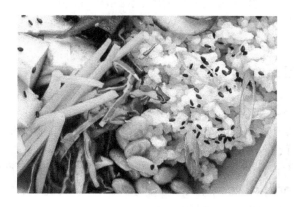

PREP TIME: 10 mins COOK TIME: 10 mins TOTAL TIME: 20 mins SERVINGS: 2

Ingredients:

- For Pan-Fried Tofu
- ⅛ onion (2 oz, 57 g)
- 1 block seared firm tofu (6.5 oz, 184 g)
- 1 Tbsp sesame oil (broiled)
- 3 Tbsp soy sauce
- ½ Tbsp rice vinegar (I utilized Mizkan Natural Rice Vinegar)
- 1 tsp stew paste (Sambal Oelek)
- For Vegan Poke Bowl
- 1 carrot (3.5 oz, 100 g)
- ¼ English cucumber (2 oz, 57 g)
- ½ watermelon radish (2.5 oz, 70 g)
- ⅛ red cabbage (3 oz, 90 g)

- 2 green onions/scallions (1 oz, 30 g)
- ½ avocado (3.5 oz, 100 g)
- 1 lime
- 2 cups cooked Japanese short-grain brown rice
- 2 Tbsp shelled edamame (1 oz)
- ½ tsp toasted dark sesame seeds
- ½ tsp toasted white sesame seeds

Directions:

1. Accumulate every one of the ingredients.
2. Veggie lover Poke Bowl Ingredients
3. To Make Pan-Fried Tofu
4. In the event that you need to serve hot tofu, begin setting up the vegetables first (look down) and return to this progression later. Something else, meagerly cut the white onion.
5. Vegetarian Poke Bowl 1
6. Open the tofu bundle and eliminate any dampness with a paper towel. Cut the tofu into scaled down pieces, around 12 pieces.
7. Veggie lover Poke Bowl 2
8. Heat sesame oil in a large skillet over medium heat and add the white onion.
9. Veggie lover Poke Bowl 3
10. Sauté until the onion is covered with oil. At that point add the tofu solid shapes.
11. Vegetarian Poke Bowl 4
12. When the tofu is covered with oil, add soy sauce, Mizkan Natural Rice Vinegar, and sambal oelek.
13. Veggie lover Poke Bowl 5
14. Lessen the heat to medium-low and coat the tofu with the sauce. Mood killer the heat and

eliminate it from the oven once the tofu is very much covered with the sauce.

15. Vegetarian Poke Bowl 6
16. To Prepare Vegetables (Toppings)
17. Julienne the carrot. Cut the carrot into slim pieces and afterward cut into julienne strips. I utilize this julienne peeler and cut down the middle longwise.
18. Vegetarian Poke Bowl 7
19. Strip the cucumber skin, leaving some part unpeeled (so it looks decent), and cut into meager cuts.
20. Vegetarian Poke Bowl 8
21. Strip the watermelon radish and cut into slim cuts.
22. Veggie lover Poke Bowl 9
23. Eliminate the extreme center of the red cabbage and daintily shred.
24. Veggie lover Poke Bowl 10
25. Corner to corner cut the green onions/scallions into dainty cuts.
26. Veggie lover Poke Bowl 11
27. Tenderly strip the avocado and cut into ½ inch cuts.
28. Veggie lover Poke Bowl 12
29. At that point cut the avocado into 3D squares. Slice the lime down the middle and press the juice over the avocado to keep it from browning.
30. Veggie lover Poke Bowl 13
31. To Assemble Vegan Poke Bowls
32. Serve the cooked brown rice in two large dishes. Spot the massive ingredients first, for example, seared tofu, avocado, and red

cabbage. At that point add the remainder of the ingredients. Sprinkle sesame seeds and green onions on top.

33. Choose what kind of tofu to utilize.

34. In the wake of attempting diverse tofu for the Vegan Poke Bowl, my family enjoyed these two sorts of pan fried tofu.

35. 2 sorts of rotisserie Tofu.

36. The rotisserie firm tofu on the left is our #1 decision for the jab bowl. It is denser than "firm" tofu. The seared outside keeps its shape as well as gives tasty exquisite flavor. When you cut it into 3D squares, within is delicate and assimilates all the delightful sauce! You can buy this sort of tofu in the refrigerated segment in customary (American) supermarkets.

37. The correct tofu is a typical fresh, singed tofu puffs that you can discover in Asian supermarkets. It can likewise be called southern style tofu squares or wipe singed tofu. These singed tofu puffs are made with fresh tofu skin that acts like a wipe. It's incredible in retaining flavors, however you may feel you're eating air as it does not have the tofu surface.

Pick An Assortment Of Beautiful Fixings

38. For a quick arrangement, I pick a rainbow scope of vegetables that are prepared to eat crude. You cut down on cooking time, however these new, fresh vegetables likewise give a pleasant difference to the delicate steamed rice and tofu. The outcome is an even, energizing bowl that is loaded with flavors and surfaces.

39. A white dishes containing flavorful sautéed tofu, cucumber, avocado, edamame, carrot, red cabbage, and watermelon radish over brown rice.

40. In this formula, I added avocado, carrot, cucumber, edamame, red cabbage, scallion, and watermelon radish. Go ahead and change around with various vegetables, for example, sunflower sprouts, instant pickles, cherry tomatoes, red radish, or mango!

Think About The Development And Structure

41. The jab bowl is intended to grandstand new ingredients and brilliant vegetables in a perfectly introduced bowl. So it merits considering how you would need to set up the vegetables or garnishes. – regardless of whether daintily cut or guilefully cubed – they ought to be effortlessly combined as one when you eat.

2.   Avocado Toast

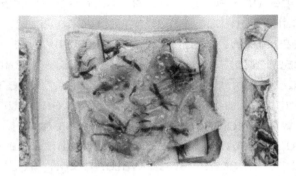

PREP TIME: 30 mins COOK TIME: 30 mins SERVINGS: 6 Avocado Toasts

Ingredients:

- 1 Basic Avocado Toast
- 1 cut shokupan (Japanese pullman portion bread)
- ½ avocado
- 1 wedge lemon
- freshly ground dark pepper
- flake ocean salt
- sesame oil (simmered)
- 2 Avocado Toast with Furikake
- 1 cut shokupan (Japanese pullman portion bread)
- ½ avocado
- 1 wedge lemon
- flake ocean salt
- sesame oil (simmered)
- furikake (rice preparing)
- 3 Avocado Toast with Japanee (Spicy) Mayo and Shichimi Togarashi

- 1 cut shokupan (Japanese pullman portion bread)
- ½ avocado
- 1 wedge lemon
- sesame oil (simmered)
- flake ocean salt
- ½ Tbsp Japanese mayo
- ½ Tbsp sriracha sauce
- shichimi togarashi (Japanese seven zest)
- 4 Avocado Toast with Ramen Egg
- 1 cut shokupan (Japanese pullman portion bread)
- ½ avocado
- 1 wedge lemon
- sesame oil (simmered)
- flake ocean salt
- ramen egg (ajitsuke tamago) (Recipe in Notes)
- roasted prepared ocean growth
- shichimi togarashi (Japanese seven zest)
- 5 Avocado Toast with Smoked Salmon
- 1 cut shokupan (Japanese pullman portion bread)
- ½ avocado
- 1 wedge lemon
- sesame oil (simmered)
- flake ocean salt
- sliced cucumber
- smoked salmon
- 2 shiso leaves (perilla/ooba)
- ikura (salmon roe)
- soy sauce
- 6 Avocado Toast with Fried Egg
- 1 cut shokupan (Japanese pullman portion bread)

- ½ avocado
- 1 wedge lemon
- freshly ground dark pepper
- flake ocean salt (This salt has delicate, sheer, pyramid-like chips, which give food a delightful look and crunchy finish. This salt will add a mind boggling, a trace of briny flavor to the food. Britain's Essex coast is the place where the most mainstream brand, Maldon, is collected.)
- sesame oil (cooked)
- cherry tomatoes (optional)
- red radish (optional)
- fried egg

Guidelines:

1. Instructions to Prepare Avocado
2. Assemble every one of the ingredients. This is for the Basic Avocado Toast. Toast a cut of Shokupan (Japanese pullman portion bread).
3. Avocado Toast Ingredients
4. Slice the avocado down the middle by running the blade around it. Wind.
5. Avocado Toast 1
6. On the off chance that you are using just a large portion of an avocado, save the one with seed for some other time. I utilize this avocado guardian to stay away from oxidation. You can likewise press lemon juice on a superficial level.
7. Avocado Toast 2
8. Smack the seed and eliminate it. Scoop the avocado tissue with a spoon.

9. Avocado Toast 3
10. Crush avocado with a fork and press the lemon. Combine all as one.
11. Avocado Toast 4
12. #1 Basic Avocado Toast
13. Move the crushed avocado onto a toasted shokupan. Press the avocado delicately to equally appropriate with a fork. Season with newly ground dark pepper and chipped ocean salt.
14. Avocado Toast 5
15. Shower sesame oil over the avocado. Serve right away.
16. Avocado Toast 6
17. #2 Avocado Toast with Furikake
18. Move the pounded avocado onto a toasted shokupan. Press the avocado delicately to uniformly circulate with a fork. Season with piece ocean salt and furikake. Shower sesame oil over the avocado. Serve right away.
19. Avocado Toast 7
20. #3 Avocado Toast with Japanese Mayo or Spicy Mayo and Shichimi Togarashi
21. Rather than pounded avocado, you can present with cut avocado. Strip the avocado skin, and cut the avocado into ¼ inch cuts.
22. Avocado Toast 8
23. Tenderly squeezed to falter and press the lemon to cover the avocado with lemon juice.
24. Avocado Toast 9
25. Move the cut avocado to a toasted shokupan, shower sesame oil over the avocado, and season with chip ocean salt.
26. Avocado Toast 10

27. To make zesty mayo, blend Japanese mayo and sriracha sauce. On the off chance that you don't care for hot mayo, basically utilize just mayo. Shower Japanese mayo or zesty mayo on top of the avocado cuts and sprinkle Shichimi Togarashi on top. Serve right away.
28. Avocado Toast 11
29. #4 Avocado Toast with Ramen Egg
30. Move the squashed avocado onto a toasted shokupan. Press the avocado delicately to equally circulate with a fork. Sprinkle sesame oil and season with piece ocean salt.
31. Avocado Toast 12
32. Cut the ramen egg (Ajitsuke Tamago) into equal parts and spot on top of the pounded avocado toast.
33. Avocado Toast 13
34. Topping with Korean ocean growth and sprinkle Shichimi Togarashi on top. Serve right away.
35. Avocado Toast 14
36. #5 Avocado Toast with Smoked Salmon
37. Move the squashed avocado onto a toasted shokupan. Press the avocado delicately to uniformly convey with a fork. Sprinkle sesame oil and season with chip ocean salt.
38. Avocado Toast 15
39. Using a peeler, meagerly cut the cucumber and eliminate abundance dampness with a paper towel. Put the cut cucumber and afterward smoked salmon on top.
40. Avocado Toast 16

41. Fold up shiso leaves and cut into julienned strips. Enhancement on top of the smoked salmon.
42. Avocado Toast 17
43. Spot some ikura and shower soy sauce on top. Serve right away.
44. Avocado Toast 18
45. #6 Avocado Toast with Fried Egg
46. Move the squashed avocado onto a toasted shokupan. Press the avocado tenderly to equally appropriate with a fork. Season with newly ground dark pepper and piece ocean salt.
47. Avocado Toast 19
48. Sprinkle sesame oil and spot some split cherry tomatoes and cut red radish.
49. Avocado Toast 20
50. Put the singed egg on top and season with piece ocean salt and newly ground dark pepper.
51. **Tips:**
52. Purchase "ready" avocado: Your supermarkets sell avocado with a "ready" sticker on avocados. Prepare them when you're to make avocado toast.
53. A crush of lemon juice: To keep the new green avocado tone, add 1 tablespoon of pressed lemon juice to half of the avocado.
54. Squash however you would prefer: I accept crushed avocado turns out best for avocado toast (than cut avocado), yet that is only my inclination. I will in general squash mine better so it's smooth and lay comfortably like a thick

coat over the hot bread. Leave it chunkier if that is the thing that you favor.

55. Toast your bread: This is really clear obviously, however ensure your bread is pleasantly toasted. Not exclusively you'd get a crunchy and hot flavor, however toasting the bread gives it a solid base to help the heaviness of avocado.

56. Shower sesame oil: If you have been sprinkling additional virgin olive oil, offer it a reprieve and attempt toasted/broiled (dim) sesame oil. It's a distinct advantage!

3. Eggplant Donburi

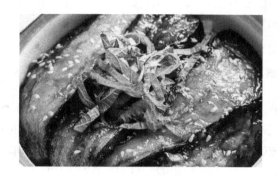

PREP TIME: 10 mins COOK TIME: 10 mins TOTAL TIME: 20 mins SERVINGS: 2

Ingredients:

- 7 oz Japanese/Chinese eggplant (2 Japanese eggplants; on the off chance that you use globe eggplant, cut into the wedges or adjusts with skin on. Skin will keep the eggplant shape while cooking.)
- 10 shiso leaves (perilla/ooba) (or utilize 1 green onion)
- 1 handle ginger
- 2 Tbsp potato starch/cornstarch
- 4 Tbsp unbiased enhanced oil (vegetable, rice grain, canola, and so forth) (isolated; utilize 2 Tbsp at a time)
- ½ tsp toasted white sesame seeds
- Flavors
- 4 Tbsp mirin (Not by and large same, however substitute with 4 tsp sugar + 4 Tbsp purpose/water; Please change the sweetness

dependent on your inclination; read more about mirin)
- 2 Tbsp soy sauce (or use GF soy sauce for sans gluten)

Guidelines:

1. Accumulate every one of the ingredients.
2. Soy Glazed Eggplant Donburi Ingredients
3. Cut eggplant into ¼ inch cuts and sprinkle salt (generally ½-1 tsp). Put away for 15 minutes and wipe off the dampness with a paper towel.
4. Soy Glazed Eggplant Donburi 1 and 2
5. Wash the shiso leaves and dry with a paper towel. Dispose of the stems.
6. Soy Glazed Eggplant Donburi 3
7. Move up the shiso leaves and cut into chiffonade strips.
8. Soy Glazed Eggplant Donburi 4
9. Strip the ginger skin and mesh the ginger. You'll require 1 tsp ginger.
10. Soy Glazed Eggplant Donburi 5
11. Put 2 Tbsp potato starch in a little plate and daintily coat the eggplant cuts on the two sides.
12. Soy Glazed Eggplant Donburi 6
13. Heat the 2 Tbsp oil in a skillet over medium heat. At the point when the oil is hot, add the eggplant cuts in a solitary layer. Cook until the base side is golden brown, around 3-4 minutes. Up to that point, don't contact the eggplants to accomplish a pleasant singe.
14. Soy Glazed Eggplant Donburi 7

15. At the point when the base side is pleasantly burned, shower the remainder of oil (2 Tbsp) on top and flip the eggplant cuts to cook the opposite side, around 3-4 minutes.
16. Soy Glazed Eggplant Donburi 8
17. When this side is cooked till golden brown, decrease the heat to medium-low heat and add mirin, soy sauce, and ground ginger.
18. Soy Glazed Eggplant Donburi 9 NEW
19. Take it back to stew and spoon the sauce over the eggplant a couple of times. In the event that the sauce got thicken excessively quick (because of the potato starch), add 1 Tbsp water at a time to loosen a piece. Eliminate from the heat when the eggplant is very much covered with the sauce.
20. Soy Glazed Eggplant Donburi 10 NEW
21. Serve steamed rice in a donburi bowl (somewhat greater than rice bowl) and shower some sauce.
22. Soy Glazed Eggplant Donburi 11
23. At that point place the eggplant cuts on top. For show, I cover each cut somewhat. Topping with shiso leaves and sprinkle sesame seeds. Serve right away.
24. **Tips:**
25. Keep the eggplant skin
26. Eggplant tissue gets delicate and delicate when it's cooked through, and on the off chance that you cook it for a really long time, the substance gets soft. In this way, it's vital to:
27. Keep the eggplant skin connected to the substance to keep up its shape.

28. Cut the eggplant so the substance is held by the skin.
29. For this reason, I just suggest using Japanese, Chinese, or Italian eggplant. On the off chance that you utilize American/glove eggplant, cut into the wedges and utilize just the part that has skin (and utilize the center part for different recipes).
30. 2. Sprinkle salt
31. Eggplant has delicate, elastic tissue with small air pockets that acts like a wipe in absorbing oil and fluids. While we like the eggplant to assimilate every one of the great flavors, the test is to keep it from getting oily.
32. The secret to that is by separating the air pockets and diminishing the elasticity by salting the eggplant first. Salting additionally keeps the eggplant from staining.
33. Simply make a point to clear off the overabundance water prior to browning.

Use Potato Starch/Cornstarch
34. Covering the eggplant with potato starch (or cornstarch) can help:
35. Keeps the eggplant from absorbing all the oil.
36. Makes a pleasant golden covering.

4. Dashi Recipe From Mushrooms

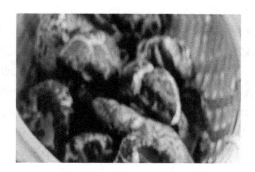

PREP TIME: 5 mins STEEPING TIME: 15 mins TOTAL TIME: 20 mins SERVINGS: 1 dashi (a bit less than ½ cup or 2 cups)

Ingredients:

- For Preparing Rehydrated Shiitake Mushrooms
- 3 dried shiitake mushrooms (They can be found in Japanese/Asian/Chinese supermarkets. The heaviness of each dried mushroom differs from 5 grams to 10 grams relying upon the size and thickness.)
- ½-⅔ cup water (enough to cover mushrooms)
- For Making Shiitake Dashi
- 3 dried shiitake mushrooms
- 2 cups water

Guidelines:

1. How to Rehydrate Dried Shiitake Mushrooms

2. Assemble every one of the ingredients. Check if there are any residue or earth caught under the gills of the mushrooms, and if there are, utilize a cake brush to clean. Try not to wash it submerged.
3. Shiitake Dashi Ingredients 1
4. In a perfect world, you need to make shiitake dashi early. Spot the mushrooms in a bricklayer container or a sealed shut compartment and pour cold water to cover the mushrooms (and wet them). Allow them to absorb the fridge for a couple of hours or ideally overnight. In any case, in the event that you are in a rush, place the mushrooms in a bowl and absorb them warm water (internal heat level) for 15 minutes or until relaxed. Put something substantial on top of the mushrooms with the goal that they will be lowered under warm water and become completely re-hydrated.
5. Shiitake Dashi 1
6. At the point when shiitake mushrooms are delicate, crush to deplete, saving the fluid.
7. Shiitake Dashi 2
8. Rehydrated shiitake mushrooms are prepared to utilize. Eliminate and dispose of the intense stem of the mushrooms with a blade. You can utilize these rehydrated shiitake mushrooms as though you utilize crude shiitake mushrooms.
9. Shiitake Dashi 3
10. Run the splashing fluid through a fine strainer (get any earth and so on) Utilize the concentrated shiitake dashi for cooking, by

including the sauce, steaming, preparing, and so on No squandering!

11. Shiitake Dashi 4
12. To Store
13. In the event that you intend to put something aside for some other time, you can store in the cooler for 2-3 days and multi month in the cooler.
14. Shiitake Dashi 5
15. How to Make Shiitake Dashi
16. Accumulate every one of the ingredients. Check if there are any residue or soil caught under the gills of the mushrooms, and if there are, utilize a cake brush to clean. Try not to wash it submerged.
17. Shiitake Dashi Ingredients 2
18. Drench the shiitake mushrooms in 2 cups water. On the off chance that you have time, let them absorb the fridge for a couple of hours or ideally overnight. In case you're in a rush, absorb them warm water for 15 minutes or until relaxed.
19. Shiitake Dashi 10
20. Subsequent to drenching for a few hours...
21. Shiitake Dashi 6
22. At the point when shiitake mushrooms are delicate, press to deplete, saving the fluid.
23. Shiitake Dashi 7
24. Rehydrated shiitake mushrooms are prepared to utilize. Eliminate and dispose of the extreme stem of the mushrooms with a blade. You can utilize these rehydrated shiitake mushrooms as though you utilize crude shiitake mushrooms.
25. Shiitake Dashi 8

26. Run the drenching fluid through a fine sifter and use it for cooking (this is the shiitake dashi).
27. Shiitake Dashi 9
28. To Store
29. On the off chance that you intend to put something aside for some other time, you can store in the cooler for 2-3 days and multi month in the cooler.
30. Tips to Get the Best Flavor from Dried Shiitake Mushrooms:
31. Great dried shiitake mushrooms are costly, however the flavors and surface are stunning.
32. Purchase thick mushrooms with profound white crevices on the cap (more flavor).
33. Utilize cold water to douse dried shiitake mushrooms to gradually draw out the flavor from mushrooms, ideally overnight.
34. To make shiitake dashi, kindly note that we can just utilize dried shiitake mushrooms on the grounds that new shiitake mushrooms don't have similar profound and serious flavors as the dried ones.

5.   Vegan Miso Soup

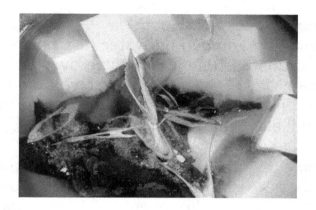

***PREP TIME: 15 mins COOK TIME: 15 mins
TOTAL TIME: 30 mins SERVINGS: 4***

Ingredients:

- For Kombu Dashi
- 4 cups water
- 1 kombu (dried kelp) (0.4 oz, 10 g; 4" x 4", 10 x 10 cm; add more for more grounded flavor)
- For Miso Soup
- 1 Tbsp dried wakame ocean growth
- 2 green onions/scallions
- 7 oz delicate/luxurious tofu (kinugoshi tofu) (½ bundle)
- 5 Tbsp miso

Guidelines:

1. Assemble every one of the ingredients.
2. Vegetarian Miso Soup Ingredients

3. Make Kombu Dashi
4. Put the kombu in 4 cups of water and let steep for 20 minutes, or as long as you can (most extreme short-term).
5. Veggie lover Miso Soup 1
6. Move the kombu and water to a pot. Welcome it to approach edge of boiling over on medium heat. On the off chance that you didn't steep for quite a while at Step 1, it's nice to gradually bring the kombu water to approach bubbling on low heat. When the air pockets begin to show up and it would appear that bubbling, eliminate the kombu and mood killer the heat. In the event that you leave the kombu in water, kombu dashi can turn out to be harsh. So it's generally prescribed to take out. Utilize this utilized kombu to make a stewed kombu or natively constructed furikake (rice preparing).
7. Veggie lover Miso Soup 2
8. Get ready Other Add-ins and Garnish
9. Rehydrate dried wakame kelp in water for 5 minutes. Crush water out and place it in miso soup bowls.
10. Veggie lover Miso Soup 3
11. Cut the green onions into little pieces (slantingly – optional) and put away in a little bowl.
12. Veggie lover Miso Soup 4
13. Set the miso soup bowls and green onion to the side until further notice.
14. Vegetarian Miso Soup 5
15. Add Miso

16. An ordinary Japanese miso soup bowl holds around 200 ml of fluid. Miso shifts in pungency relies upon types and brands; however when in doubt, we add 1 tablespoon (20 g) of miso per one miso soup bowl (200 ml dashi). I use miso muddler (one side estimates 1 Tbsp, the opposite side 2 Tbsp). For this formula, I utilize about 4-5 Tbsp. Tip: When you add tofu, you might need to add an additional tablespoon (that is the reason I add 5 Tbsp absolute) since tofu contains extra dampness which weakens miso soup.
17. Veggie lover Miso Soup 6
18. At the point when you add miso, turn off the heat (we should NEVER allow miso to soup bubble). Scoop some dashi/soup into your spoon and let the miso break down in the scoop first using chopsticks or a whisk. Tip: Do not straightforwardly drop miso into the soup since you may wind up with undissolved pieces of miso left in the soup. It's vital to taste to check the pungency.
19. Vegetarian Miso Soup 7
20. Add Tofu
21. Cut tofu into little 3D shapes and add to the miso soup (Please utilize a cutting board on the off chance that you are not used to cutting it on your palm).
22. Vegetarian Miso Soup 8
23. Reheat until hot (however not bubbling) and serve. Tip: After adding miso, never let miso soup bubble (It will lose the fragrance and flavor and furthermore execute the probiotics in the miso.)

6. Spinach With Sesame Miso Sauce

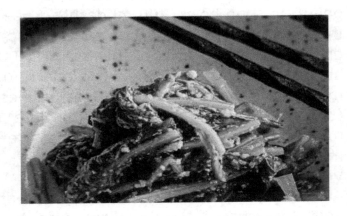

PREP TIME: 10 mins COOK TIME: 5 mins TOTAL TIME: 15 mins SERVINGS: 4 (as a small side)

Ingredients:

- ¼ tsp fit/ocean salt (I use Diamond Crystal; utilize half for table salt)
- 6 oz spinach
- Sesame Miso Sauce
- 1 Tbsp mirin
- 2 Tbsp toasted white sesame seeds
- 2 tsp miso (I utilized Hikari Miso® Organic Koji Miso)
- 1 tsp sugar
- ½ tsp soy sauce

Guidelines:

1. Assemble every one of the ingredients. Heat a major pot of water to the point of boiling. [Optional] If your sesame seeds are not toasted/cooked at this point, or in the event that you need more hot taste/aroma, put sesame seeds in a griddle and toast them on low heat. At the point when 2-3 sesame seeds begin to fly from the skillet, eliminate from the heat.
2. Spinach with Sesame Miso Sauce Ingredients
3. While trusting that the water will bubble, add 1 Tbsp mirin in a little pot. Cook it over medium heat until the liquor is dissipated, approximately 30 seconds. Put away.
4. Spinach with Sesame Miso Sauce 1
5. In a suribachi (mortar), add 2 Tbsp sesame seeds and pound with a surikogi (pestle) until sesame seeds are nearly ground. It's ideal to leave some surface.
6. Spinach with Sesame Miso Sauce 2
7. Add 2 tsp miso, 1 tsp sugar, liquor free mirin, and ½ tsp soy sauce and combine well as one.
8. Spinach with Sesame Miso Sauce 3
9. When water is bubbling, add the salt. Hold the spinach leaves so you can begin whitening from the stem (which takes more time to cook). Cook for 15 seconds. Give up the verdant part and cook for 30 seconds.
10. Spinach with Sesame Miso Sauce 4
11. Eliminate spinach from the water and absorb frosted water to stop the cooking. On the other

hand, channel and run the spinach under chilly running water until cool.

12. Spinach with Sesame Miso Sauce 5
13. Gather the spinach and press water out.
14. Spinach with Sesame Miso Sauce 6
15. Cut the spinach into 2" (5cm) lengths and add to the bowl.
16. Spinach with Sesame Miso Sauce 7
17. Combine the spinach and sauce as one. Serve at room temperature or chilled.
18. Spinach with Sesame Miso Sauce 8
19. To Store
20. You can place it in a water/air proof holder and store it in the cooler for 2-3 days or in the cooler for 2 a month.

7. Spinach And Feta Turnovers

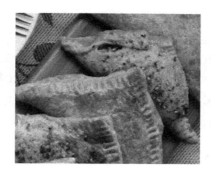

***PREP TIME: 15 mins COOK TIME: 30 mins
TOTAL TIME: 45 mins SERVINGS: 6 Turnovers***

Ingredients:

- 1 tsp extra-virgin olive oil
- ¼ cup onion (finely chopped)
- 3 cloves garlic (minced)
- 7 oz spinach leaves
- kosher/ocean salt (I use Diamond Crystal; utilize half for table salt) (for taste)
- freshly ground dark pepper (for taste)
- 1 tsp lemon juice
- 1 large egg (50 g w/o shell) (isolated)
- 3 oz feta cheddar (disintegrated)
- 12 oz frozen puff baked good (thawed out)
- Za'atar (optional; this is a Middle Eastern and North African zest mix most ordinarily comprised of a blend of dried thyme, oregano, marjoram, sumac, and sesame seeds. It is accessible at forte food shops in the US and

can be requested from online zest shops like The Spice House and Penzeys Spices.)

Guidelines:

1. Heat the olive oil in a large skillet over medium heat. Add the onion and garlic and cook until just relaxed (be mindful so as not to consume the garlic). Add the spinach and cook, blending regularly, until completely withered, around 3 minutes.
2. Eliminate from the heat. Season gently with salt and pepper and overwhelmingly mix in the lemon squeeze and egg yolk (hold the egg white for some other time). Move the combination to a bowl and permit to cool.
3. When the spinach is sufficiently cool to deal with, press out however much fluid as could reasonably be expected and generally slash. (I understand that it appears to be nonsensical to place fluid in then crush it out, however after endless trials this cycle prompted the best outcomes.) Return spinach to the bowl and altogether blend in the feta.
4. Preheat the oven to 400°F (200ºC). For a convection oven, decrease cooking temperature by 25ºF (15ºC). Line a preparing sheet with material paper.
5. Carry out the puff baked good to a square shape about ⅛ inch (3 mm) thick and 12" x 18" (30 x 46 cm). Cut into 6 even 5"- 6" (13-15 cm) squares. Put a spoonful of the spinach-feta combination into the focal point of each puff cake square. Crease the puff baked good

over to shape a triangle. Press down with a fork along the edges to firmly seal.

6. Move the turnovers to the readied heating sheet. Brush with the saved egg white and sprinkle with za'atar, if using. Put in the oven and heat for 20 minutes, or until golden brown.

7. Spinach and Feta Turnovers 2

8. Eliminate from the oven and permit to cool marginally prior to serving. Spinach-feta turnovers are amazing warm or at room temperature.

9. To Store

10. The turnovers can be made ahead and frozen. To freeze, lay level on a preparing plate and put in the cooler. Once frozen, move to cooler packs. To re-heat, just prepare in a pre-heated oven for 10 to 15 minutes, until warmed through.

8. Spinach Salad With Asian Salad Dressing

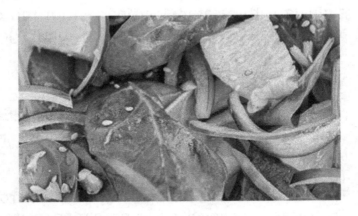

PREP TIME: 10 mins TOTAL TIME: 10 mins SERVINGS: 2

Ingredients:

- 3 Tbsp simmered pecans
- ¼ red onion
- 1 navel orange
- 3 oz infant spinach
- Dressing
- 3 Tbsp nonpartisan enhanced oil (vegetable, rice wheat, canola, and so forth)
- 2 Tbsp soy sauce
- 1½ Tbsp rice vinegar
- ¼ tsp ground ginger
- ¼ tsp sugar
- ½ Tbsp toasted white sesame seeds
- ⅛ tsp newly ground dark pepper
- ¼ tsp genuine/ocean salt (I use Diamond Crystal; utilize half for table salt)

Guidelines:

1. To make the dressing, in a little bowl, whisk together 3 Tbsp vegetable oil, 2 Tbsp soy sauce, 1 ½ Tbsp rice vinegar, ¼ tsp ground ginger, ¼ tsp sugar, and ½ Tbsp sesame seeds and put away.
2. Spinach Salad 1
3. Heat a griddle over medium high heat and toast the pecans, blending often until fragrant. Move the pecans to a plate and put away.
4. Spinach Salad 2
5. Cut the red onion meagerly. Cut the navel orange into 8 wedges. Cut off the strip and essence. Cut each wedge into 2-3 pieces.
6. Spinach Salad 3
7. Add the spinach, the navel orange, and pecans in a large bowl. Pour as much dressing as you like and throw tenderly to cover altogether. Serve right away.
8. **Tips:**
9. Here are a few ideas of ingredients you could place in your dressing combination:
10. Salt and Freshly Ground Black Pepper is a MUST: Adding a touch of salt draws out the genuine kind of the food, actually like a sorcery. Rather than adding more flavors, add a touch of salt to change. On the off chance that you are using pungent ingredients like soy sauce, make sure to diminish the measure of salt added.

11. New Ingredients: Chop garlic, ginger, shallots, chives, parsley and scallions into fine pieces and add them into the dressing.
12. Flavors: Dijon mustard, mayonnaise, soy sauce, ponzu, miso, tahini, red pepper chips, ground sesame seeds, and so forth... You can add nearly anything!
13. Sweeteners: Don't be hesitant to sweeten if the corrosive part is excessively solid. You can add nectar, sugar, brown sugar, maple syrup, agave nectar, and so forth
14. New or Dried Herbs: Choose one of spices like basil, oregano, marjoram, mint, dill, and so forth to add more flavors.
15. Sprinkles: Sprinkle sesame seeds, pecans, almonds, pine nuts, walnuts, cashews to add surface to the dressing and salad!

9. Spinach Salad With Sesame Dressing

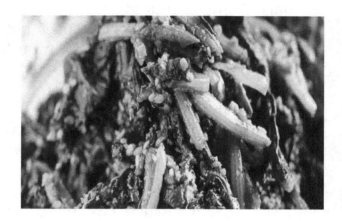

PREP TIME: 10 mins COOK TIME: 5 mins TOTAL TIME: 15 mins SERVINGS: 4

Ingredients:

- ½ lb spinach
- 1 tsp fit/ocean salt (I use Diamond Crystal; utilize half for table salt) (for whitening spinach)
- Sesame Sauce
- 3 Tbsp toasted white sesame seeds
- 1 Tbsp soy sauce
- 1 Tbsp sugar
- Sesame Sauce (for grown-ups)
- 3 Tbsp toasted white sesame seeds
- 1 ½ Tbsp soy sauce
- 1 Tbsp sugar
- ½ tsp purpose
- ½ tsp mirin

Guidelines:

1. Assemble every one of the ingredients.
2. Spinach Gomaae Ingredients
3. [Optional] For the sesame sauce, put sesame seeds in a griddle and toast them on low heat. At the point when 2-3 sesame seeds begin to fly from the dish, eliminate from the heat.
4. Spinach Gomaae 2
5. Granulate the toasted sesame seeds with a mortar and pestle. Leave some sesame seeds unground for some surface.
6. Spinach Gomaae 1
7. Add the sesame sauce flavors to the ground sesame seeds and combine all as one.
8. Spinach Gomaae 2
9. Put delicately salted water in a large pot and bring to bubble. When bubbling, add the spinach from the stem side (takes more time to cook) and cook for 30-45 seconds. Tip: American spinach is delicate and we can eat it crude not at all like Japanese spinach; subsequently, cooking for 30-45 seconds is sufficient.
10. Spinach Gomaae 3
11. Eliminate the spinach from the water and absorb frosted water to quit cooking with residual heat. Then again, channel and run the spinach under chilly running water until cool. Gather the spinach and crush water out.
12. Spinach Gomaae 4
13. Cut the spinach into 1-2" (2.5-5 cm) lengths and put in a medium bowl.

14. Spinach Gomaae 5
15. Add the sesame sauce and throw it all together. Serve at room temperature or chilled.
16. Spinach Gomaae 6
17. To Store
18. You can keep the extras in a water/air proof compartment and store in the cooler for 2-3 days or cooler for 2 a month.

10.   Mashed Tofu Salad

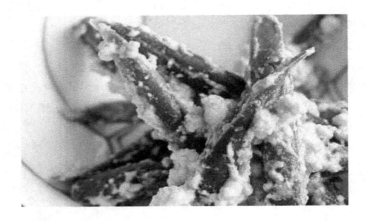

***PREP TIME: 10 mins COOK TIME: 5 mins
DRAINING TIME: 15 mins TOTAL TIME: 30 mins
SERVINGS: 2***

Ingredients:

- 7 oz medium tofu (momen tofu) (½ block)
- 9 oz green beans
- Flavors
- 4 Tbsp toasted white sesame seeds
- 1 Tbsp sugar
- 2 tsp miso (I use Hikari Miso® Organic White Miso)
- 1 tsp soy sauce
- ⅛ tsp fit/ocean salt (I use Diamond Crystal; utilize half for table salt)

Guidelines:

1. Assemble every one of the ingredients. To store the extra tofu, keep it in a sealed shut holder and pour water until it covers the tofu. Keep in the cooler (change the water each day) and use it inside a couple of days.
2. Green Bean Shiraae Ingredients
3. To Prepare Tofu
4. Try not to avoid this progression. You would prefer not to empty the water out of tofu totally, however it's imperative to eliminate some dampness so the dressing doesn't get excessively wet. Wrap the tofu with paper towels.
5. Green Bean Shiraae 1
6. Put the wrapped tofu on a plate or plate. Add another plate or plate on top of the tofu and put a hefty article on top to work with depleting. Put away for 30 minutes.
7. Green Bean Shiraae 2
8. To Prepare Green Beans
9. Heat a major pot of water to the point of boiling. Detach the closures of green beans.
10. Green Bean Shiraae 3
11. Bubble green beans until fresh delicate (kindly don't overcook).
12. Green Bean Shiraae 4
13. Channel well and put away.
14. Green Bean Shiraae 5
15. Cut the green beans askew into 2-inch (5 cm) pieces.
16. Green Bean Shiraae 6

17. Pour the soy sauce and throw together. Put away for some other time.
18. Green Bean Shiraae 7
19. To Prepare Sesame Seeds
20. Toast the sesame seeds in a griddle, shaking the container every now and again, until they are fragrant and begun to pop. Move to a Japanese mortar (suribachi).
21. Green Bean Shiraae 8
22. Granulate sesame seeds with a pestle (surikogi).
23. Green Bean Shiraae 9
24. To Make Tofu Dressing
25. Add sugar and miso.
26. Green Bean Shiraae 10
27. Blend well until sugar and miso are consolidated into the ground sesame seeds.
28. Green Bean Shiraae 11
29. Eliminate tofu from the paper towel. Break it into pieces with your hands and add to the sesame seed combination.
30. Green Bean Shiraae 12
31. Using a pestle, squash and pound the tofu until smooth or however you would prefer.
32. Green Bean Shiraae 13
33. It's critical to taste the tofu and season with salt to taste. It ought not be tasteless. Green beans will be added, so the tofu dressing ought to have great flavor at this stage.
34. Green Bean Shiraae 14
35. Combine all as one until smooth.
36. Green Bean Shiraae 15
37. To Assemble

38. Make certain to shake off any abundance soy sauce from the green beans first. Any fluid from the soy sauce will just weaken the dressing. At that point add the prepared green beans to the tofu dressing. Consolidate well.
39. Green Bean Shiraae 16
40. Once joined, you can chill in the fridge for 30 minutes prior to serving, or serve right away.
41. Green Bean Shiraae 17
42. To Store
43. You can save it for 24 hours in the cooler; notwithstanding, I suggest devouring it soon.
44. **Tips:**
45. Channel tofu
46. It's interesting the amount you should deplete your tofu, however you can generally make the change each time.
47. You would prefer not to weaken your dressing with abundance water from the tofu. Simultaneously, you would prefer not to eliminate the water totally as sodden tofu adds delicate surface to the dish.
48. To discover the equilibrium, I normally channel for 15-30 minutes. In the event that I need to abbreviate to 15 minutes, I would put something weighty on top of the tofu to work with the depleting cycle. On the off chance that I have 30 minutes, I would not put any weight and let it channel normally.
49. 2. Toast the sesame seeds
50. Indeed, the greater part of the sesame seeds sold in bundles are as of now toasted. Be that as it may, you can toast it again in the griddle to draw out the more aroma.

51. 3. Utilize white miso
52. For the rich tofu dressing, I like to utilize White Miso (Shiro Miso 白味噌) in light of the fact that the shading and sweet flavor supplement the combination. Here's one from Hikari Miso® Organic White Miso that I utilized in this formula.
53. Hikari Miso® Organic White Miso
54. Hikari Miso has been my go-to miso for longer than 10 years. You can discover Hikari Miso® items in your nearby Japanese supermarkets and Asian business sectors.
55. 4. Crush the tofu till smooth and rich
56. Except if you favor a stout tofu surface, I prescribe to streamline the blend until satiny. At the point when cooled, the pounded tofu gives a pleasant reviving taste and it's scrumptious!
57. 5. Season the vegetables with soy sauce prior to blending
58. Make certain to prepare the whitened vegetables with soy sauce first. Thusly, you can shake off any abundance fluid prior to adding them to the tofu blend.

11. Broccolini Gomaae

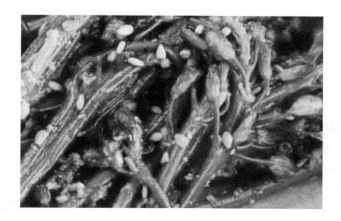

PREP TIME: 5 mins COOK TIME: 10 mins TOTAL TIME: 15 mins SERVINGS: 4

Ingredients:

- ½ lb broccolini
- ⅛ tsp fit/ocean salt (I use Diamond Crystal; utilize half for table salt)
- 3 Tbsp toasted white sesame seeds
- 1 Tbsp soy sauce
- 1 Tbsp sugar

Directions:

1. Accumulate every one of the ingredients.
2. Broccolini Gomaae Ingredients
3. Wash the broccolini in running water, cut and dispose of the closures.
4. Broccolini Gomaae 1

5. Heat a large pot of water to the point of boiling. When bubbling, add a touch of salt and put the finish of broccolini first into the bubbling water and afterward lower the remainder of broccolini. Bubble for 2 minutes.
6. Broccolini Gomaae 2
7. Eliminate the broccolini and absorb the frosted water to cool.
8. Broccolini Gomaae 3
9. Get a couple of lots of broccolini and press the water out. Spot them in a perfect bowl.
10. Broccolini Gomaae 4
11. Add the sesame seeds in a large griddle and toast them until a couple of sesame seeds begin flying, about 1.5 minutes. Throw the skillet while toasting so sesame seeds will not get scorched.
12. Broccolini Gomaae 5
13. Move the toasted sesame seeds into a Japanese-style pestle and furrowed mortar and continue to granulate until the surface gets smooth.
14. Broccolini Gomaae 6
15. Add sugar and soy sauce to squashed sesame seed and blend well.
16. Broccolini Gomaae 7
17. Blend the sesame sauce with the broccolini and serve at the room temperature or chilled.
18. Broccolini Gomaae 8
19. To Store
20. You can keep the extras in an impermeable compartment and store in the fridge for as long as 3 days and in the cooler for 3 weeks.

12. Soy Milk Hot Pot

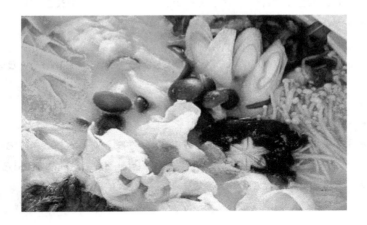

PREP TIME: 20 mins COOK TIME: 20 mins TOTATIME: 40 mins SERVINGS: 4

Ingredients:

- 7 oz enoki mushrooms (1 bundle)
- 3.5 oz shimeji mushrooms (1 bundle)
- 4 shiitake mushrooms
- ¼ napa cabbage (1.5 lb, 680 g)
- ½ bundle mizuna (Japanese mustard green) (or spinach or any salad greens)
- 1 pack shungiku (Tong Ho/Garland Chrysanthemum) (or any mixed greens)
- 1 negi (long green onion) (or leek or green onions/scallions)
- 1 green onion/scallion
- 1 medium tofu (momen tofu) (14 oz, 396 g)
- ½ daikon radish (1 lb, 454 g)
- 1 carrot (3 oz, 85 g)
- 1 gobo (burdock root) (5.3 oz, 150 g)
- Hot Pot Soup

- 3 cups dashi (Japanese soup stock; snap to find out more) (720 ml) (I use Awase dashi. Kombu dashi for veggie lover/vegetarian)
- ¼ cup purpose (4 Tbsp)
- ¼ cup mirin (4 Tbsp)
- 2 cups unsweetened soy milk (microwave till it's warm)
- ¼ cup miso (4 Tbsp; I use awase miso)
- 2 Tbsp toasted white sesame seeds
- ¼ tsp legitimate/ocean salt (I use Diamond Crystal; utilize half for table salt) (to taste)
- Plunging Sauce
- ponzu

Guidelines:

1. Assemble every one of the ingredients.
2. Soy Milk Hot Pot (Tonyu Nabe 豆乳鍋) | EasJapanese Recipes at JustOneCookbook.com
3. To Prepare Hot Pot Broth
4. In your donabe (stoneware pot) or a large pot, add 3 cups (720 ml) dashi, ¼ cup (60 ml) purpose, and ¼ cup (60 ml) mirin. Cover and heat the soup to the point of boiling on medium heat.
5. Soy Milk Hot Pot 1
6. When bubbling, add 2 cups (480 ml) warm soy milk. On medium heat, gradually heat up until the soup nearly bubbles. Keep the top uncovered and mix sometimes. Then, pound 2 Tbsp toasted sesame seeds in a pestle and mortar.
7. Soy Milk Hot Pot 2

8. When the soup is hot, add ¼ cup (4 Tbsp) miso and ground sesame seeds.
9. Soy Milk Hot Pot 4
10. Taste the soup and add genuine salt in the event that you like it saltier. Relies upon the brands and kinds of miso, the pungency of your soup will fluctuate. I suggest making the soup somewhat saltier since you'll add vegetables that will deliver water and weaken the soup. Mood killer the heat and put away. Keep it covered.
11. Soy Milk Hot Pot 5
12. Hot Pot Ingredients: If your meat isn't daintily cut, you need to cut it meagerly all alone. Perceive how to do it (picture is daintily cut hamburger).
13. Instructions to Slice Meat 7
14. Cut off and dispose of the lower part of enoki mushrooms and shimeji mushrooms.
15. Soy Milk Hot Pot 5-a
16. Cut off and dispose of the shiitake stem. In the event that you like, make an improving cut on shiitake mushrooms.
17. Soy Milk Hot Pot 6
18. Cut napa cabbage into 2" (5 cm) pieces widthwise. At that point cut into 2-3 pieces the long way on the thick and white base piece of napa cabbage so that it'll be quicker to cook.
19. Soy Milk Hot Pot 7
20. Cut Mizuna (or spinach) and shungiku into 2" (5 cm) pieces.
21. Soy Milk Hot Pot 8-a

22. Cut negi (long green onion or leek) into 1" (2.5 cm) thick pieces askew. Meagerly cut green onion/scallion.
23. Soy Milk Hot Pot 8-b
24. Cut the tofu block into 1" (2.5 cm) cuts.
25. Soy Milk Hot Pot 10
26. Using a vegetable peeler, strip the daikon and carrot meagerly as though you are stripping their skin. You can cut these root vegetables into meagerly adjusts or quarters, yet my family adores eating root vegetables in long paper-slender structure.
27. Soy Milk Hot Pot 11
28. Strip the gobo (burdock root) same path as daikon and carrot. Splash the daintily cut gobo in water for 15 minutes to keep them from evolving shading.
29. Soy Milk Hot Pot 12
30. Put every one of the vegetables, mushrooms, and tofu in a platter.
31. Soy Milk Hot Pot 13
32. Begin cooking a portion of the extreme/thick vegetables (the intense piece of napa cabbage leaves, negi, tofu, mushrooms, daikon, carrot, and gobo) over medium heat, saving some for later cluster just as the verdant vegetables that will cook quick. Cover the top so it will cook quicker. When the stock is stewing, decrease the heat to medium-low heat so the stock will not coagulate. Stew for 10 minutes, however ensure you will not allow it to bubble. You can either begin serving food that is cooked. Root vegetables set aside a more extended effort to cook. Add the meat and

verdant vegetables and cover to cook until the meat is not, at this point pink. Using a fine-network skimmer, skim any sours gliding on the soup. You can eat the turn sour or dispose of it.

33. Soy Milk Hot Pot 14
34. To Eat
35. Every individual ought to have a little bowl of ponzu sauce and chopped scallions. Plunge the cooked meat and vegetables in ponzu sauce to enjoy! Continue to cook the ingredients in the pot as you enjoy the dinner.
36. To Store
37. You can keep the extras in a hermetically sealed compartment and store in the cooler for as long as 2 days and in the cooler for as long as a month.

13. Cabbage And Onion Torta

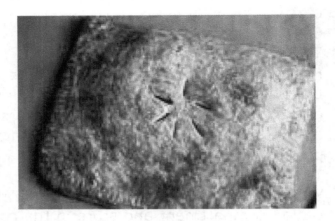

YIELD6 to 8 servings TIME1 hour 45 minutes

INGREDIENTS:

- 475 grams generally useful flour (4 cups)
- 60 grams entire wheat flour (1/2 cup)
- 12 grams genuine salt (around 2 1/2 teaspoons), more depending on the situation
- 12 tablespoons unsalted margarine, chilled and cubed
- ¼ cup olive oil, more depending on the situation
- 1 large Spanish onion, divided and cut (2 1/2 cups)
- 1 ½ pounds Savoy or customary cabbage (1 little head), cored and cut
- Dark pepper, depending on the situation
- 2 teaspoons juice vinegar, or to taste
- ⅓ cup dry bread pieces

- 5 large garlic cloves, finely chopped
- 1 ½ tablespoons thyme leaves
- 8 ounces fontina cheddar, ground (2 cups)
- 2 ounces diced smoked ham like bit (optional)
- 1 large egg yolk
- Add to Your Grocery List
- Fixing Substitution Guide
- Wholesome Information

Planning:

1. To make the cake, consolidate flours and 7 grams (1/2 teaspoons) salt in a large bowl. Using a cake shaper or two forks, cut in margarine until it structures coarse morsels. Add 1 to 1/2 cups freezing water, working it in a couple of tablespoons all at once, until combination simply meets up. Structure batter into a ball, cover with plastic, and refrigerate for in any event 1 hour or overnight.
2. Heat 2 tablespoons oil in a large skillet over medium-high heat. Add the onion and cook, blending every so often, until delicate and softly browned, around 10 minutes.
3. Add 1 tablespoon oil and mix in cabbage, a modest bunch at a time, waiting for every option to shrink marginally prior to adding more. Season with 5 grams (1 teaspoon) salt and some pepper. Cook until cabbage is delicate and any fluid has vanished, around 7 to 10 minutes. Mix in vinegar and cook until dissipated, scraping up any browned pieces from the lower part of the skillet. Move combination to a bowl. Taste and add more

salt, vinegar or both, depending on the situation.

4. Add staying 1 tablespoon oil to skillet and mix in bread pieces, garlic and thyme. Cook until bread pieces start to shading, around 1 moment. Scratch into a bowl.

5. Heat oven to 425 degrees. Oil a large heating sheet.

6. On a floured surface, carry out mixture into a 17-by-12-inch square shape. Move to the heating sheet. With the long side confronting you, spread a large portion of the bread pieces equally over right 50% of mixture, leaving a 1/2-inch line. Top with a large portion of the cheddar, at that point cover cheddar with a large portion of the cabbage combination. Rehash layers. Sprinkle ham over the top whenever wanted.

7. Touch edges of mixture with water. Overlay left half over filling and utilize the prongs of a fork to seal edges. Brush hull with egg yolk. Using a blade, cut a few cuts in the focal point of the top outside layer. Move pie to oven and heat until covering is golden brown and firm, 40 to 50 minutes. Cool for at any rate 15 minutes prior to cutting and serving. Serve warm, or reheat prior to serving.

8. **Tip**

9. Estimations for dry ingredients are given by weight for more prominent precision. The same estimations by volume are inexact.

14. Croatian Sarma Recipe (Stuffed Cabbage Rolls)

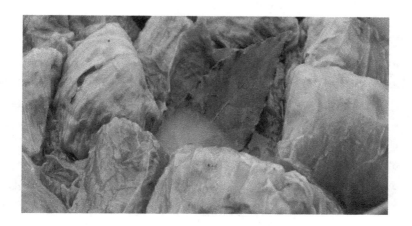

Prep time: 30 min Cook time: 15 min

Ingredients:

- Sarma
- Whole cured cabbage head
- 1 kg of mincemeat (2.2 lbs). I favor half pork neck and half veal, yet you can utilize whatever you like best
- 200 g of finely diced špeck or smoked bacon (8 oz)
- 4 stripped and squashed garlic cloves
- 1/2 pack generally chopped parsley leaves
- 3 Tbls. of pop water or a major touch of bicarbonate pop
- 1 cup of uncooked rice
- 1/2 Tbls. Vegeta

- 1 Tbls. hot ground paprika (optional)
- 1 Tbls. sweet paprika (optional)
- 2 Tbls. breadcrumbs (optional)
- Salt and pepper to taste
- 1 egg
- 1 Tbls. olive oil
- Sarma Sauce
- 2 onions, chopped fine
- 3 Tbls. additional virgin olive oil
- 100 g diced smoked špeck/pancetta or smoked bones (4 oz)
- 1/2 pack chopped parsley
- 2 carrots diced little
- 400 g (little tin) passata (2 cups)
- 1/2 kg shredded sauerkraut (3 cups). Ensure you give it an awesome wash in new water prior to using
- Salt and pepper

Guidelines:

1. Sarma Preparation
2. Take a whole salted cabbage head. You'll track down these on Amazon or in European shops in the chilled area. Wash each leaf altogether. Eliminate the thick piece of the stem without tearing the leaves. It's ideal to permit the leaves to deplete on some paper towel or wipe every unique case
3. Take a large blending bowl, and consolidate mincemeat, bit, garlic, parsley leaves, soft drink water or bicarbonate pop, rice, Vegeta, hot paprika (optional), sweet paprika

(optional), breadcrumbs (optional), Salt and pepper, egg and olive oil

4. Blend the entirety of the ingredients until very much joined
5. How about we Roll The Sarma
6. You need every one of the leaves to be about the very size so that each cabbage move cooks simultaneously. So feel free to slice any large leaves down the middle, and furthermore combine two more modest leaves as you go
7. Take approx 3 tablespoons of the minced meat, and delicately consolidate in the palm of your hand. Try not to roll or pack as this will make them too thick when you eat them
8. Spot the meat on the edge of the cabbage leaf and roll away from you. At that point wrap up the sides of the leaf tenderly into the meat. There ought to be no uncovered meat. On the off chance that there is, eliminate a portion of the filling
9. Put the sarma away, and set up the sauce
10. Sarma Sauce
11. In a shallow pan, or stunningly better, a Le Creuset cast-Iron dish, sprinkle in some additional virgin olive oil, add the 2 diced onions and cook until straightforward on low heat. At that point add the 2 diced carrots, diced spot, and parsley. Keep on singing on low heat until carrots begin to mollify
12. Add the shredded sauerkraut and make a layer on the lower part of the pot. Presently, pack the Croatian sarma into the pot. They ought to be pressed near one another.

13. Pour in bubbling water with the goal that it simply covers the sarma. Add the passata and a spot of salt and pepper. At regular intervals, give the pot a shake (don't mix them or they will break) and allow them to stew for 2 hours on a low-medium heat

14. Notes

15. Never blend in with a spoon as you will break the arms. Continuously shake the pot or utilize a spoon to delicately move them.

15. Easy Carrot Salad

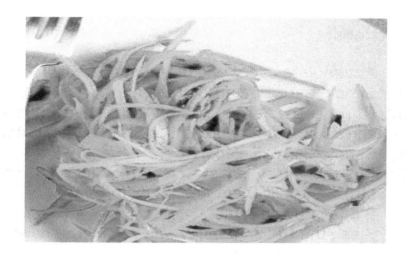

PREP TIME: 15 mins CHILL TIME: 1 hr TOTAL TIME:
1 hr 15 mins SERVINGS: 4 (as a side)

Ingredients:

- 2 carrots (10 oz, 280 g)
- 1 twig Italian parsley
- Flavors
- ¼ tsp legitimate/ocean salt (I use Diamond Crystal; utilize half for table salt)
- freshly ground dark pepper
- 2 Tbsp extra-virgin olive oil
- 1 Tbsp lemon squeeze (or rice vinegar)
- ¼ tsp sugar (optional; add in the event that you use rice vinegar)
- Optional (Only on the off chance that you like to add)
- ¼ tsp Dijon mustard (blend in with flavors)

- roasted pecans (sprinkle)
- raisins (sprinkle)

Directions:

1. Accumulate every one of the ingredients.
2. Simple Carrot Salad Ingredients
3. Using a peeler, strip the carrot into flimsy sheets, and afterward cut them in equal parts.
4. Simple Carrot Salad 1
5. Cut the flimsy sheets of carrots into julienne strips and put them in a medium bowl.
6. Simple Carrot Salad 2
7. Slash the Italian parsley and add to the bowl.
8. Simple Carrot Salad 3
9. Add every one of the flavors (½ tsp salt, newly ground dark pepper, 2 Tbsp olive oil, and 1 Tbsp lemon juice).
10. Simple Carrot Salad 4
11. Allow them to marinate for at any rate 1 hour prior to serving. The carrot salad will save for 5-6 days in the cooler.

16. Boiled Large Pumpkin Puree

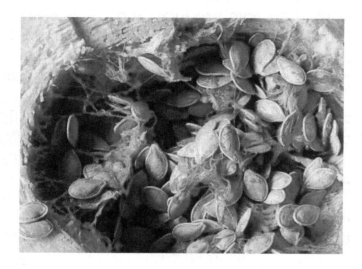

Yield: Yield will depend on size and meatiness of the pumpkin Time: Active Time: 30 min | Inactive Time: 45 min total

Ingredients:

- 1 large pumpkin—anything greater than a foot and gauging in excess of 7 pounds
- Scraps, Wilts + Weed

Directions:

1. A large Halloween pumpkin, proposed for cutting, for the most part has just 2 creeps of tissue. All things considered, it yields a lot of goodness. For example, a 8-pound (2-foot-distance across) pumpkin can deliver sufficient

puree for three pies, in addition to seeds, which can be caramelized for a debauched tidbit. However, cooking it can introduce difficulties. It tends to be hard to cut up a large stringy organic product, and it's precarious to fit it in a little oven. So I suggest the accompanying methodology.

2.   With a hefty knife, remove the lower part of the pumpkin; hold for Layered Pumpkin Pie. Slash the remainder of the pumpkin into 5-inch pieces. Scoop out the seeds and put away to broil later (see Caramelized Roasted Pumpkin Seeds).

3.   In a large pot over high heat, join the pumpkin lumps and 5 cups water. Heat to the point of boiling, lessen the heat, and stew for 45 minutes, until relaxed. Channel. In groups, puree the pieces in a food processor until coarsely smooth, around 3 minutes. Refrigerate for a couple of days in a shut compartment or measure and freeze in clumps for as long as a half year.

17. Creamy Miso Pasta With Tofu And Asparagus

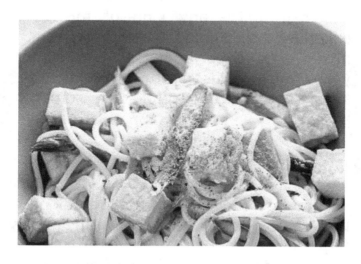

PREP TIME: 5 mins COOK TIME: 15 mins TOTAL TIME: 20 mins SERVINGS: 2

Ingredients:

- For Pasta
- 1 seared firm tofu (6.5 oz, 184 g)
- 4 oz asparagus
- 1 Tbsp extra-virgin olive oil
- ¼ tsp legitimate/ocean salt (I use Diamond Crystal; utilize half for table salt)
- freshly ground dark pepper
- For Cooking Spaghetti
- 1 ½ Tbsp genuine/ocean salt (I use Diamond Crystal; utilize half for table salt)
- 7 oz spaghetti
- Soy Milk Sauce

- ½ cup unsweetened soy milk (twofold the sum in the event that you need to make it soup pasta)
- 2 tsp miso (twofold the sum for soup pasta; you can utilize any kind of miso with the exception of Hatcho Miso - white miso is milder, red miso is bolder and saltier, and yellow miso (Awase Miso) is in the middle)
- 1 tsp soy sauce (twofold the sum for soup pasta)

Directions:

1. Accumulate every one of the ingredients.
2. Rich Miso Pasta with Tofu and Asparagus Ingredients
3. To Make Miso Soymilk Sauce/Soup
4. In an estimating cup, consolidate ½ cup soy milk, 2 tsp miso, and 1 tsp soy sauce, and combine all as one. On the off chance that you need to make it into a "soup pasta" (see my blog entry), twofold the measure of these ingredients.
5. Smooth Miso Pasta with Tofu and Asparagus 8
6. To Prepare Pasta Ingredients
7. Wrap the tofu with a paper towel and eliminate any dampness. Cut the tofu into little 3D squares (It would be simpler to eat in the event that you cut the tofu into more modest blocks).
8. Velvety Miso Pasta with Tofu and Asparagus 1 and 2Creamy Miso Pasta with Tofu and Asparagus 1 and 2

9. Trim off the closures of asparagus and cut it slantingly into flimsy cuts.
10. Velvety Miso Pasta with Tofu and Asparagus 3
11. To Cook Spaghetti
12. Begin bubbling 4 quarts (16 cups, 3.8 L) water in a large pot (I utilized a 4.5 QT Dutch oven). When bubbling, add 1 ½ Tbsp salt and spaghetti.
13. Rich Miso Pasta with Tofu and Asparagus 4
14. Mix to ensure spaghetti doesn't adhere to one another. Tip: I as a rule decrease the cooking time by 1 moment on the off chance that I need to keep cooking the pasta subsequently. Channel on the off chance that you wrap up cooking the spaghetti first, yet you ought to have the option to cook the remainder of the ingredients shortly while spaghetti is being cooked.
15. Rich Miso Pasta with Tofu and Asparagus 5
16. To Cook Pasta
17. Heat the olive oil in a large skillet over medium heat. Add tofu solid shapes and saute until they are covered with oil and warm.
18. Rich Miso Pasta with Tofu and Asparagus 6
19. Add asparagus and season with salt.
20. Rich Miso Pasta with Tofu and Asparagus 7
21. Add the soy milk combination to the dish and lower the heat to medium-low heat (to abstain from turning sour).
22. Rich Miso Pasta with Tofu and Asparagus 9
23. Hold 4 Tbsp (¼ cup, 60 ml) of pasta water and add to the skillet. On the off chance that you are making the "soup pasta", add 4 more Tbsp of pasta water here.

24. Velvety Miso Pasta with Tofu and Asparagus 10
25. At this point, your spaghetti ought to be done (something else, turn off the heat and trust that spaghetti will get done with cooking). Get the noodles with a couple of utensils (or you can rapidly deplete in the sink) and add to the dish. Increment the heat to medium and throw the spaghetti to combine all as one.
26. Smooth Miso Pasta with Tofu and Asparagus 11
27. Taste and add salt if necessary. The saved pasta water I added has sufficient salt so I don't add extra salt here. Serve the pasta to singular dishes. Sprinkle with Shichimi Togarashi in the event that you like a kick of flavor. Enjoy!

Conclusion

I would like to thank you for choosing this book. It contains alkaline diet recipes which are healthy and can prevent you from certain diseases. Also, these recipes will help you in weight reduction. Prepare and enjoy.

ALKALINE COOKBOOK MADE EASY FOR BEGINNERS

Table of Contents

INTRODUCTION

Groundbreaking Benefits of Following an Alkaline Diet:

Battles against Fatigue: Too much corrosive in the body diminishes the stock of oxygen. This reductions the cell's capacity fix and gather supplements. On the off chance that you feel languid and tired for the duration of the day, even with the legitimate measure of rest, this could be the pointless development of corrosive.

Fortifies Immune System: Unbalance in pH diminishes the body's capacity to battle microscopic organisms and infections. Without the oxygen, microorganisms and infections can flourish the most in the circulatory system. Alkalizing is a need to dispense with the likelihood of illness.

Diminishes aggravation: Over-acridity in the body can build irritation, when you have coronary illness, joint pain, or disease your framework is in a fiery state. A diet that comprises of alkaline-framing food sources holds aggravation under tight restraints.

Reinforces Bone: As individuals age, the body normally goes through calcium from our bones Calcium in a critical factor in adjusting the blood and body pH. Without the calcium, our bones become fragile, prompting osteoporosis.

18. Tofu Pudding

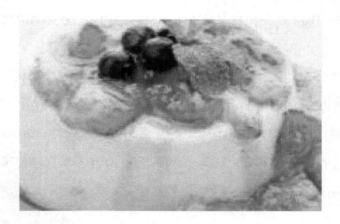

PREP TIME: 20 mins CHILLING TIME: 1 hr TOTAL TIME: 1 hr 20 mins SERVINGS: 5

Ingredients:

- ⅓ cup bubbling water
- 4 sheets gelatin sheet(s)/powder (0.4 oz, 10 g)
- 6.2 oz firm luxurious tofu
- 5 Tbsp nectar
- 1 ½ cup unsweetened soymilk
- ½ tsp almond remove
- Strawberry Sauce
- ½ lb strawberries
- 1 Tbsp nectar
- Juice from ¼ lemon
- mint leaves (for decorate)
- Extra berries (for decorate)

Guidelines:

1. Assemble every one of the ingredients. You'll require five 4-oz (120 ml) ramekins.
2. Tofu Pudding Ingredients
3. Join bubbling water and gelatin in a bowl (or estimating cup) and whisk together until gelatin is totally disintegrated.
4. Tofu Pudding Blancmange
5. Cut tofu into 1 inch blocks and add them inside a food processor. Gather nectar and soymilk and puree all into a single unit.
6. Tofu Pudding Blancmange
7. Move the blend to a large bowl. Add the gelatin blend and almond concentrate and speed without making a lot bubbles.
8. Tofu Pudding Blancmange
9. On the off chance that you like your pudding to have additional smooth surface, run the combination through a fine cross section strainer (optional).
10. Tofu Pudding Blancmange
11. Scoop the combination into singular ramekins. Chill in the fridge until set, for in any event 60 minutes.
12. Tofu Pudding Blancmange
13. In the mean time make the strawberry sauce. Cut strawberries into little 3D squares and pound with fork or potato masher. Add nectar and lemon juice.
14. Tofu Pudding Blancmange
15. At the point when the pudding is set, run a blade around the pudding to slacken. Turn over

onto a plate and shake delicately to deliver the pudding. Pour the strawberry sauce and trimming with mint leaves and additional berries (assuming any) on top.

16. Tofu Pudding Blancmange
17. To Store
18. You can save the extras in the cooler for as long as 3 days.

19. Fruit Granola

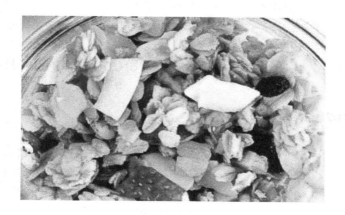

PREP TIME: 10 mins COOK TIME: 30 mins COOLING TIME: 1 hr TOTAL TIME: 1 hr 40 mins SERVINGS: 8 cups

Ingredients:

- 3 cups older style moved oats (Use 4 cups on the off chance that you avoid puffed rice; No substitute with different sorts of oats. You need to utilize antiquated moved oats for this formula to get the correct granola surface.)
- 2 cups puffed rice (I utilized Crisp Rice Cereal from Trader Joe's)
- 1 ½ cup crude nuts or potentially seeds (I utilized ½ cup (65 g) pumpkin seeds, ½ cup (55 g) walnuts, ½ cup (50 g) cut almonds. In the event that all around simmered, add in after the granola is cool.)
- 1 tsp legitimate/ocean salt (I use Diamond Crystal; utilize half for table salt)
- ½ cup coconut oil (softened, or olive oil)

- ½ cup maple syrup (or nectar)
- 1 cup dried and freeze-dried organic products (I utilized blend of raisins, dried apricot, dried peach, freeze-dried strawberries and freeze-dried apples)
- ¼ cup coconut drops (crude or broiled)

Guidelines:

1. Assemble every one of the ingredients. Preheat the oven to 350ºF (180ºC) and place the oven rack in the middle. For a convection oven, decrease cooking time by 25ºF (15ºC). Line a rimmed half-sheet heating dish with material paper.
2. Simple Homemade Granola Ingredients
3. In a large blending bowl, add the oats, puffed rice, genuine salt, and unroasted nuts and seeds (walnuts, cut almonds, and pumpkin seeds). In the event that your nuts and seeds are broiled, blend in after the granola is totally cool.
4. Simple Homemade Granola 1
5. Mix to mix along with a silicone spatula. In the event that you will add flavors (or other dry ingredients), you can add now before wet ingredients so you can mix well.
6. Blending granola and nuts in a metal blending bowl
7. Pour in the coconut oil and maple syrup and blend well until everything is very much covered.
8. Simple Homemade Granola 3

9. Move the granola onto your readied heating dish. With the rear of the silicone spatula, spread it in an even layer and press down the granola.
10. Simple Homemade Granola 4
11. Heat at 350ºF (180ºC) for 12-15 minutes (We will prepare an aggregate of 25-30 minutes) and eliminate the container from the oven.
12. Simple Homemade Granola 5
13. Mix to get an even shading and ensure the granola is cooking equally. Press down the granola with the rear of the spatula to make an even layer. In the event that you utilize crude coconut chips, add them during the most recent 10 minutes of preparing.
14. Simple Homemade Granola 6
15. Set the heating skillet back in the oven, and keep on preparing for another 12-15 minutes, or until gently golden/brown and hot. Eliminate the skillet from the oven and let the granola cool totally on a wire rack, generally for 60 minutes. The granola will keep concocting and firm during this time so don't contact it.
16. Simple Homemade Granola 7
17. Then, hack the dried products of the soil dried natural products into little pieces.
18. Simple Homemade Granola 8
19. At the point when the granola is COMPLETELY cool, top with the dried products of the soil dried organic products (counting my simmered coconut pieces). Break the granola into pieces with your hands (I like to keep greater lumps).
20. Simple Homemade Granola 9

21. Store the granola in water/air proof containers or holders at room temperature for 7-10 days. You can likewise freeze them for as long as 2 months.
22. Tips to make Homemade Fruit Granola
23. Here are my tips for accomplishing the best custom made granola:
24. Sweetener and oil proportion ought to be balanced: The covering for your granola ought to be one section sweetener and one section oil.
25. Use material paper: It will help the sweetener adheres to your oats and make it simple to move the granola whenever it's finished.
26. To get huge clumpy stout granola: you should 1) put the oats a little swarmed in the container so they can stay together, 2) press the granola down into an even layer with a spatula prior to placing into the oven, and 3) mix it just once partially through cooking.
27. Don't overbake: Although you need your granola to be pleasantly toasted, remove it from the oven when it looks LIGHTLY toasted/golden on top and scents decent. Granola will dry and get crunchy as it cools.
28. Allow the granola to cool totally: Do not touch or split it up to that point.
29. A white bowl containing custom made granola with blackberries.

20. Steamed Vegetables With Miso Sesame Sauce

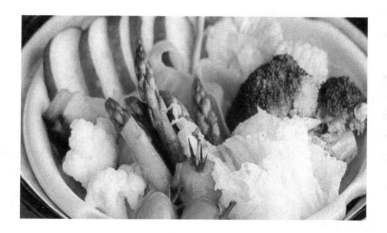

PREP TIME: 20 mins COOK TIME: 10 mins TOTAL TIME: 30 mins SERVINGS: 4 people (as side dish)

Ingredients:

- 2 cups dashi (I utilized the standard awase dashi (kombu + katsuobushi) for steaming vegetables, however for veggie lover/vegan, use kombu dashi or water)
- Vegetables for Steaming (change as you like)
- 1 Japanese sweet potato (Satsumaimo)
- ½ gobo (burdock root)
- ¼ kabocha (squash/pumpkin)
- 1 carrot
- 1 ear new corn
- 10 asparagus
- 1 head broccoli
- 1 head cauliflower

- 5 leaves napa cabbage
- 10 cherry tomatoes
- Miso Sesame Sauce
- 6 Tbsp toasted white sesame seeds
- 2 cloves garlic
- 1 tsp sugar
- 2 Tbsp miso
- 2 Tbsp soy sauce
- 2 Tbsp sesame oil (cooked)
- 4 Tbsp mirin
- 2 Tbsp rice vinegar
- ¼ tsp genuine/ocean salt (I use Diamond Crystal; utilize half for table salt)

Directions:

1. To Prepare the Miso Sesame Sauce
2. Assemble every one of the ingredients for Miso Sesame Sauce.
3. Steamed Vegetables Ingredients 1
4. Granulate 6 Tbsp sesame seeds with a pestle and mortar.
5. Steamed Vegetables 1
6. Pulverize 2 cloves garlic. Add 1 tsp sugar and 2 Tbsp miso and consolidate well.
7. Steamed Vegetables 2
8. Add 2 Tbsp soy sauce, 2 Tbsp sesame oil, 4 Tbsp mirin, and 2 Tbsp rice vinegar. Blend well.
9. Steamed Vegetables 3
10. Check the taste and add genuine salt if vital. I added ¼ tsp salt.
11. Steamed Vegetables 4
12. To Prepare the Vegetables

13. Set up every one of the ingredients. Make dashi; something else, use water all things being equal.
14. Steamed Vegetables Ingredients 2
15. Cut the sweet potatoes into ¼ inch cuts (uniform more modest pieces will cook quicker than larger parts) and absorb water to eliminate starch. Channel and put away.
16. Steamed Vegetables 5
17. Wash the gobo truly well and strip it daintily with a peeler. Absorb water promptly to keep away from shading changes and change the water once. Channel and put away.
18. Steamed Vegetables 6
19. Dispose of the seeds from kabocha and cut daintily.
20. Steamed Vegetables 7
21. You can either cut the carrot into ¼ inch cuts or utilize a peeler to strip the carrot.
22. Steamed Vegetables 8
23. Cut the natural corn into 1-inch thickness.
24. Steamed Vegetables 9
25. Hold every asparagus, snap and dispose of the more limited base end. Slice the asparagus down the middle.
26. Steamed Vegetables 10
27. Cut the broccoli and cauliflower into florets.
28. Steamed Vegetables 11
29. Cut the napa cabbage into scaled down pieces.
30. Steamed Vegetables 12
31. To Steam
32. Pour the dashi in your liner, cover the top, and welcome it to bubble on medium-high heat. As a speedy guide, dashi (or water) ought to be in

any event 1-2 creeps to your liner (pot). Supplement the liner container. Ensure the outside of the dashi (or water) isn't contacting the crate. On the off chance that it is, take out some water.

33. Steamed Vegetables 13
34. At the point when steam is coming out from the pot firmly, decrease the heat to medium and spot the hard vegetables, for example, sweet potatoes and root vegetables. I likewise added kabocha squash and corn here as the remainder of ingredients are genuinely quick to cook. Cover the pot and set clock for 5 minutes.
35. Steamed Vegetables 14
36. At that point add "Bloom" vegetables like asparagus, broccoli, cauliflower, and the base piece of the napa cabbage. I additionally added carrot strips here. Set the clock for 3 minutes.
37. Steamed Vegetables 15
38. Finally, add the verdant piece of the napa cabbage and small scale tomatoes. Cook for 2 additional minutes.
39. Steamed Vegetables 16
40. Supplement a bamboo stick to check the doneness of denser vegetables. On the off chance that it goes through, it's prepared to eat! Stop the steaming when the vegetables are still a piece crunchy since the leftover heat will keep on cooking the vegetables.
41. Steamed Vegetables 17
42. Serve the steamed vegetables with Miso Sesame Sauce and enjoy! During the supper, you can keep on steaming the vegetables.

Watch out for the dashi/water inside the pot. Ensure you are not running out of dashi/water. On the off chance that it's excessively little, add more dashi/water.

43. Tips.

44. to Make Perfectly Steamed Vegetables
45. Utilize a large pot with the top
46. It's in every case better to utilize a greater pot where steam can circumvent the vegetables.
47. Add 1-2 cups water
48. You'll require at any rate 1 inch deep of water, barely to steam the vegetables. You can utilize the extra water for cooking. Truth be told, we use dashi – Japanese stock – to make dashi-implanted steam to cook the vegetables in this formula.
49. Add vegetables in the wake of bubbling
50. It's critical to add the vegetables after the water is totally bubbling. In the event that you add the vegetables while the water presently can't seem to heat up, the recently made steam will turn around into water beads when it contacts cold vegetables. Thus, vegetables will get more watery. In this manner, add the vegetables when there is a lot of steam coming out from the liner.
51. Keep on medium high heat
52. You need to ensure heaps of steam is ceaselessly being made, and your heat setting ought to be on medium-high. At the point when you add the vegetables, the temperature will drop rapidly, so save the heat on high for 2-3 minutes first.
53. Utilize a bamboo stick to check doneness

54. Try not to depend on the cooking time to such an extent. Indeed, even with similar vegetables, steaming time can be diverse dependent on how you cut the vegetables. The most ideal path is to utilize a bamboo stick and check whether it goes through.

21. Blueberry Pie With Cinnamon Pastry

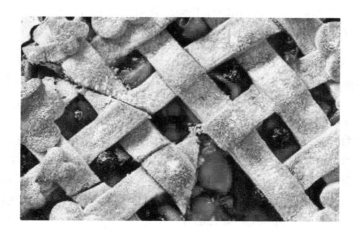

1:20 Prep 0:50 Cook 12 Servings.

INGREDIENTS:

- 4 large Granny Smith apples, cored, stripped, daintily cut
- 1/3 cup (75g) caster sugar
- 1 lemon, zested, squeezed
- 1 tsp ground cinnamon
- 1/2 tsp vanilla bean paste
- 1 cup (150g) new or frozen blueberries
- 1 tbsp cornflour
- 1 Coles Australian Free Range Egg white, daintily whisked
- 1 tbsp caster sugar, extra
- Twofold cream or vanilla frozen yogurt, to serve
- CINNAMON PASTRY

- 2 1/4 cups (335g) plain flour
- 1/2 cup (80g) icing sugar blend
- 1 tsp ground cinnamon
- 185g chilled spread, chopped
- 2 Coles Australian Free Range Egg yolks
- 1 tbsp chilled water

Strategy:

1. To make the cinnamon baked good, place flour, icing sugar, cinnamon and spread in a food processor and cycle until blend takes after fine breadcrumbs. Gather egg yolks and water and cycle until mixture comes into a single unit. Transform onto a gently floured surface and shape into a circle. Cover with cling wrap and spot in the refrigerator for 30 mins to rest.
2. Save 33% of the cake. Carry out excess cake on a gently floured surface to a 3mm-thick circle. Line the base and side of a 22cm fluted tart tin, with removable base, with cake. Trim the edge. Spot in the ice chest for 30 mins to rest.
3. In the mean time, preheat oven to 200°C. Spot the apple, sugar, lemon zing, lemon juice, cinnamon and vanilla in a pan over medium heat. Cook, mixing at times, for 5 mins or until apple begins to mellow. Add blueberries. Sprinkle with cornflour. Cook, mixing periodically, for 5 mins or until apple is delicate and juices thicken somewhat. Eliminate from heat. Put away to cool.
4. Line the baked good case with preparing paper and load up with cake loads or rice. Prepare for

10 mins. Eliminate the paper and loads or rice. Prepare for a further 8 mins or until cake is dry to the touch and light golden.

5. Spoon the apple combination into the cake case. Carry out held cake on a daintily floured surface to a 3mm-thick circle. Cut a large portion of the baked good into 2cm x 25cm strips. Organize the cake strips, slicing to fit, in a cross section design over the apple blend. Utilize heart-formed cutters to cut hearts from the leftover held baked good. Organize around the edge of the pie. Gently brush baked good with the egg white and sprinkle with additional sugar.

6. Heat for 20 mins or until cake is light golden. Put away for 5 mins to cool marginally. Cut into wedges and serve warm or at room temperature with cream or frozen yogurt.

22. Gnocchi With Pumpkin And Whipped Ricotta

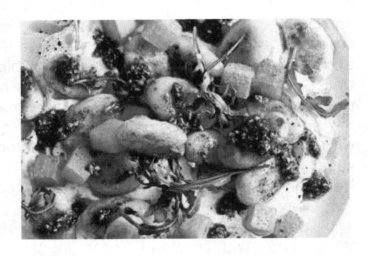

0:15 Prep 0:30 Cook 4 Servings Easy

Ingredients:

- 800g butternut pumpkin, stripped, cultivated, finely chopped
- 250g smooth ricotta
- 100g goat's cheddar
- 1/4 cup (60ml) thickened cream
- 1 amount Basic Potato Gnocchi
- 1 tbs olive oil
- 120g infant rocket leaves
- PISTACHIO PESTO
- 1/3 cup (45g) pistachios, toasted
- 2 garlic cloves, chopped
- 1/2 cup basil leaves

- 60g infant rocket leaves
- 1/4 cup (20g) finely ground parmesan
- 1/2 cup (125ml) olive oil

Technique:

1. Preheat oven to 200°C. Line a large heating plate with preparing paper. Mastermind the pumpkin on the plate and shower with olive oil splash. Season. Prepare, turning every so often, for 30 mins or until the pumpkin is golden brown and delicate.
2. Then, to make the pistachio pesto, place the pistachios, garlic, basil, rocket and parmesan in a food processor. Cycle until finely chopped. With the engine running, add the oil in a dainty, constant flow until all around consolidated. Season. Move to a little bowl.
3. Cycle the ricotta, goat's cheddar and cream in a perfect food processor until all around consolidated. Season.
4. Cook one-fourth of the gnocchi in a large pan of bubbling water for 2-3 mins or until the gnocchi ascend to the outside of the container. Utilize an opened spoon to move to a preparing plate fixed with heating paper. Rehash, in 3 bunches, with the excess gnocchi.
5. Heat oil in a skillet over high heat. Add gnocchi and cook, turning sometimes, for 2-3 mins or until golden brown. Eliminate from heat. Overlap in the pumpkin and a large portion of the pesto.

6. Spoon ricotta blend onto serving plates. Top with the gnocchi blend and sprinkle with rocket. Sprinkle with the leftover pesto.

23. Nutmeg

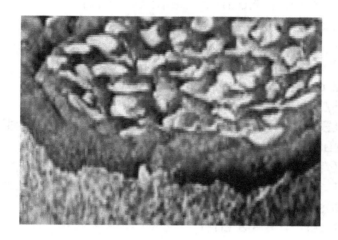

Prep time: 30 min Cook time: 40 min

Ingredients:

- Nazook: For the Pastry Dough:
- 1/2 to 2 1/2 cups universally handy flour , filtered
- 1/4 tsps dynamic dry yeast
- 1/2 cup yogurt thick
- 100 gm margarine relaxed (room temperature)
- For the Filling:
- 1/4 cup universally handy flour , filtered
- 1/4 cup sugar granulated
- 1/4 cup semolina (rawa)
- 1/4 cup almonds coarsely powdered (I powdered chipped)
- 75 gm margarine relaxed (room temperature)
- 3 to 4 cases cardamom , powdered
- 2 tbsps yogurt for brushing the baked goods

- 2 to 3 tbsps sesame seeds toasted white (optional) For the Pastry Dough :
- Armenian Nutmeg Cake With Cashewnuts
- 1 cup milk
- 1 tsp heating pop
- 2 cups universally handy flour
- 2 tsps heating powder
- 1/2 cups brown sugar , freely packeds
- 150 gm margarine cold , ideally unsalted , cubed
- 1/3 cup cashewnut pieces
- 1 to 1/2 tsps nutmeg ground , as indicated by tastes
- 1 tsp masala chai

Guidelines:

1. You can do this by hand however I utilized the processor to ply the mixture. To make the baked good batter, place 1/2 cups of the filtered flour and the dry yeast in the processor bowl and heartbeat on more than one occasion to blend. Add the yogurt and margarine and cycle into a mixture. Whenever required continue to add an as much flour as required and ply into a delicate versatile batter that is barely shy of tacky.
2. Cover the mixture and refrigerate for 3-5 hours, or overnight as you like. I wound up refrigerating the mixture for very nearly 36 hours!
3. At the point when prepared to make the baked goods take the batter out and keep at room temperature for around 10 to 15 minutes to

mollify it marginally. In the in the interim make the filling by placing every one of the ingredients for the filling into a bowl and combining as one till it looks clumpy and sand-like.

4. To make the Naazook, partition the mixture into 2 parts. Delicately work the batter so it smooth. Residue your functioning surface delicately with flour and fold the mixture into a large square shape. It ought to be slender yet not straightforward.

5. Spread a large portion of the filling uniformly as close as conceivable to the edges on the short sides, keeping some of cake batter uncovered (around 1/2 u201c) along the long edges. From one of the long sides, start gradually rolling the mixture across. Be mindful so as to ensure the filling stays equitably dispersed.

6. Move right across until you have a long, meager log. Pat it down the log so it straightens out a piece. Brush the top and favors yogurt and sprinkle with sesame seeds. Softly pat them into the batter. Utilize a blade or a crease shaper to cut the sign into 10 or 12 bits of equivalent width.

7. Spot the pieces on ungreased treat sheets and prepare at 180C (350F) for around 30 minutes or till the highest points of the baked goods become golden brown. Cool totally on a wire rack. This formula makes 20 to 24 Naazook.

8. These are best eaten somewhat warm from the oven. Nazook will keep in a sealed shut holder

at room temperature a long time or can be frozen in a sans air sack for upto 3 months.

9. Armenian Nutmeg Cake With Cashewnuts

10. You can combine the cake as one by hand however I took the path of least resistance and utilized my processor. Blend the preparing soft drink into the milk and put it away. Put the flour, the preparing powder and sugar into the processor bowl and multiple times to blend well.

11. Add the spread solid shapes and run the processor till the combination takes after pretty much uniform morsels. Take half of this and press it down, using your fingers, into a covering in a 8u201d cake tin with a removable base/spring structure cake tin. I pushed down a portion of the blend at the edges as well.

12. To the excess combination in the processor, add the milk-preparing soft drink blend, the ground nutmeg and the chai masala and run till you have a smooth batter. Empty this batter into the cake tin with the squeezed outside layer.

13. Throw the cashewnut pieces in a tsp of flour till covered and sprinkle them tenderly over the outside of the batter. Heat the cake at 180C (350F) for around 35 to 45 minutes till the top is a golden brown or till a stick pushed through the focal point of the cake confesses all.

14. Cool the cake in the tin, and afterward eliminate. Cut and serve. It is best eaten while still warm.This formula makes 12 servings.

15. This cake will keep (covered) at room temperature for 2-3 days or freeze in a fixed sack for upto 3 months.

24. Cheese And Vegetable Frittata With Fruit Salad

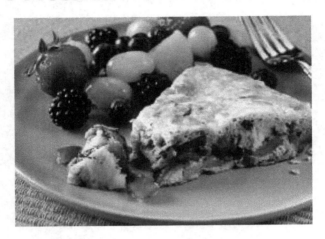

Prep time: 30 Cook time: 20

Ingredients:

- Servings
- 6
- For the Cheese and Vegetable Frittata:
- 6 large eggs
- 2 tablespoon entire wheat flour
- 1 teaspoon preparing powder
- 1/4 teaspoon dark pepper
- 1 medium onion (around 1 cup), cut into 1/2 inch pieces
- 1 cup new or frozen spinach, cut into 1/2-inch pieces
- 1 cup red as well as green chime pepper, cut into 1/2-inch pieces
- 1 cup new mushrooms
- Or on the other hand

- 1 cup canned mushrooms
- 1 clove garlic (finely chopped)
- 2 tablespoon new basil leaves (finely chopped)
- 1/3 cup part-skim mozzarella cheddar (shredded)
- Cooking splash
- For the Fruit Salad:
- 2 stripped oranges, cut down the middle, at that point into 6-8 pieces, contingent upon their size
- 1 cup new green, red or purple grapes (use assortments without seeds), left entirety
- 1 cup new or frozen strawberries, if new eliminate green top, cut into equal parts or quarters relying upon their size
- 1 cup new or frozen blended berries (blueberries, blackberries and additionally raspberries)
- 2 tsp balsamic or white wine vinegar OR new or packaged lime or lemon juice OR pineapple or potentially squeezed orange
- 2 teaspoon olive oil
- 2 Tbsp mint or basil leaves, left entire, taken out from stems

Directions:

1. Tip: Click on advance to check as finish.
2. For the Cheese and Vegetable Frittata:
3. Preheat oven (ordinary or toaster) to sear setting.
4. In a large bowl, whisk eggs together until frothy, mix in the entire wheat flour, dark pepper, and preparing powder.

5. Using a hefty skillet with an ovenproof handle, cover the skillet with cooking splash and heat on medium.
6. Add the onion and cook until it begins to get delicate, at that point add the spinach, chime pepper and mushrooms and cook for 2-3 minutes more.
7. Add the garlic and basil and cook for 1 moment. Mix to try not to consume these.
8. Add the egg combination into the dish and mix to blend the vegetables in with the eggs.
9. Cook for 5-6 minutes or until the egg blend has set on the base and starts to set on top.
10. Add the shredded cheddar and using the rear of the spoon, push gently under the eggs, so it will not consume in the oven.
11. Spot container into the oven and cook for 3-4 minutes until golden and feathery.
12. Eliminate from container, cut into 6 servings and serve.
13. For the Fruit Salad:
14. In a large bowl join all organic product salad ingredients.
15. In a little covered container shake the vinegar or juice with the olive oil to blend.
16. Add dressing to the products of the soil to cover. In the event that using frozen organic product throw delicately to try not to split them up something over the top.
17. Trimming with the new spices, if accessible.
18. Present with the frittata.
19. (See Cooking Tips for extra fixing ideas)
20. **Fast Tips**

21. Tip: For additional zest you can offer individuals paprika or dried red stew powder to add to their organic product salad. This can make the plate of mixed greens pretty zesty over the long run, so it's ideal to add just prior to eating and that way extras don't get excessively hot. This is especially acceptable with citrus natural products (oranges, grapefruit), mango and pineapple.

22. Tip: You can likewise add broccoli, eggplant or zucchini, slice into ½ inch pieces to the vegetables you put in the frittata. Your youngsters can help set out the ingredients, and relying upon their age, help break and whisk the eggs, cut the vegetables and shred the cheddar.

23. Tip: You can utilize new or frozen defrosted mango, new or canned in its own juice pineapple, new or frozen peaches, nectarines or melons, contingent upon what is season or all the more effectively accessible. When using canned natural product, pick organic product that is pressed in water, its own juice or light syrup (channel and flush).

25. Spinach Ravioli With Ricotta Cheese Filling, In Tomato Cream Sauce

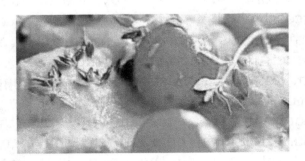

Prep Time 1 hr Cook Time 30 mins Total Time 1 hr 30 mins Ingredients

Ingredients:

- The most effective method to make ravioli batter without any preparation:
- 1/4 cups flour
- 1 egg
- 1/4 cup high temp water
- 1/4 teaspoon salt
- Spinach and ricotta cheddar ravioli filling:
- 1 tablespoon olive oil
- 10 oz spinach
- 1/2 cup Parmesan cheddar shredded
- 3/4 cup ricotta cheddar
- 1/4 teaspoon salt
- Tomato cream sauce:
- 1 tablespoon olive oil
- 2 tomatoes

- 2 garlic cloves
- 5 twigs new thyme
- 1/4 cup white wine
- 1/2 cup substantial cream
- 2 cups grape tomatoes yellow and red
- 1/4 teaspoon salt

Directions:

1. Make ravioli mixture without any preparation:
2. Blend flour in with salt.
3. Mix water with egg until very much blended.
4. In a bowl, join flour and egg-water blend together and blend until very much fused. Manipulate the mixture until well-finished and firm. The mixture ought not be excessively wet or excessively tacky. It should just adhere to itself, however not to your hands. Nonetheless, it ought not be excessively dry, all things considered. Make the mixture into a ball, cover with saran wrap. Allow the mixture to represent 1 hour at room temperature prior to using. This permits gluten to work.
5. Instructions to make ravioli cheddar filling:
6. Heat olive oil on medium heat, add spinach and cook covered, mixing infrequently, until spinach shriveled, around 15 minutes.
7. Cook for 5 or 10 additional minutes revealed until all fluid dissipates.
8. Cleave cooked spinach finely and move to a bowl. Add Parmesan cheddar and ricotta cheddar, salt to taste and blend well. Add more salt if essential.

9. The most effective method to collect ravioli using ravioli form:
10. After the ravioli batter has been resting at room temperature for 60 minutes, partition the ravioli mixture (guidelines on the best way to make ravioli mixture without any preparation are above) into 2 equivalent parts and fold every half into an exceptionally flimsy sheet with a moving pin. Make a point to have flour close by and dust the functioning surface or moving container when important, on the grounds that the batter will be tacky. It's significant that the ravioli batter be moved meagerly (paper-slight), in any case ravioli will be excessively strong when cooked, on the grounds that mixture extends during cooking. Additionally it will be truly difficult to utilize the ravioli shape if the batter isn't sufficiently meager.
11. When you moved sheets of batter, shape singular raviolis. To shape ravioli, I utilize an extremely convenient gadget, ravioli form/plate, which works incredible! Bit by bit photographs are over the formula box.
12. Here is the means by which to utilize Ravioli form:
    1) dust the functioning plate with flour
    2) lay a slim layer of cake on the plate
    3) press in the openings
    4) fill the openings with the filling, without stuffing
    5) cover with another layer of ravioli mixture, which should lay level right across the form

      6) using the moving pins or your fingers, press, close and cut the ravioli

      7) upset the plate to allow the ravioli to come out

13. At the point when you are finished molding ravioli, carry a major pot of water to bubble, add ravioli and cook for 5 minutes, at that point channel. Or then again, on the other hand, freeze ravioli until you're prepared to cook them.

14. The most effective method to make tomato cream sauce:

15. Heat olive oil in a dish over medium heat. Cleave 2 tomatoes and garlic and add to the skillet. Cook covered for around 10 minutes until tomatoes mellow.

16. Add white wine and chopped thyme. Bring to bubble and cook revealed for 5 additional minutes until half of fluid dissipates. Eliminate from heat, let it cool for a piece.

17. At that point move to blender and puree the tomato combination. Move the puree back to the container, reheat to medium heat and add hefty cream. Mix until all around joined.

18. Slice every grape tomato down the middle and add every one of them to the container with the tomato cream sauce. Salt to taste and more chopped thyme if necessary. Cook for 5 additional minutes.

19. To serve, add cooked ravioli to the sauce without a second to spare. Permit both ravioli and the sauce accomplish same temperature. When serving on plates, embellish with thyme.

20. **Formula Notes**

21. The formula for ravioli batter makes enough to make mixture for 12 raviolis, using the shape (ravioli shape makes 12 ravioli).

26. Eggplant Rollatini

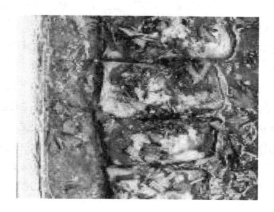

***Prep: 45 mins Stand: 15 mins Cook: 45 mins
Total: 1 hr 45 mins Yield: 16 rolls***

Ingredients:

- 4 medium eggplants
- Salt and pepper
- ¼ cup olive oil
- 1 10-oz. box frozen chopped spinach, defrosted, crushed dry
- 3 cups part-skim ricotta
- 3 cloves garlic, minced
- 2 large eggs, beaten
- 1 ½ cups shredded part-skim mozzarella
- ¾ cup ground Parmesan
- 1 24-oz. container marinara sauce

Guideline:

1. Cut closures off eggplants. Cut eggplants the long way into 1/4-inch-thick cuts, disposing of

strip covered finishes. You ought to get about 16 cuts all out. Lay cuts on a rimmed preparing sheet and sprinkle the two sides generously with salt. Let represent 15 minutes, at that point flush salt off under chilly running water and wipe cuts off.

2. Preheat oven to 400ºF. Brush the two sides of eggplant cuts with olive oil and spot in single layers on 2 heating sheets. Cook for 15 minutes, until delicate, becoming eggplant cuts over part of the way through. Let cool on sheets on wire racks until adequately cool to deal with.

3. In a large bowl, consolidate spinach, ricotta, garlic, eggs, 1/2 cup mozzarella and 1/2 cup Parmesan. Season with 1 tsp. salt and 1/2 tsp. pepper. Fog a 9-by-13-inch preparing dish with cooking splash. Spread 1/2 cup of sauce over lower part of dish. Split ricotta combination between eggplant cuts, using around 1/3 cup for each, spreading it down the middle. Move up cuts and spot crease side down in preparing dish. Top with outstanding sauce and sprinkle with residual mozzarella and Parmesan.

4. Cover preparing dish with thwart and heat for 30 minutes. Eliminate thwart and heat until browned and rising, around 15 minutes longer. Let cool for 10 minutes prior to serving.

27. Sri Lankan Dhal Curry(Parippu, Dal, Daal).

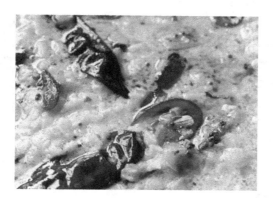

PREP TIME 10 minutes COOK TIME 20 minutes TOTAL TIME 30 minutes

Ingredients:

- Treating ingredients for dhal curry
- 3 tablespoons of oil
- A twig of curry leaves(a not many to be utilized for hardening and half while cooking the dhal)
- 4 units of garlic(a not many to be utilized for hardening promotion half while cooking the dhal)
- 1 large onion(a not many to be utilized for treating and half t while cooking the dhal)
- A teaspoon of Turmeric powder(half to be utilized for treating and half while cooking the dhal)

- 1 teaspoon of red chilies specks or two entire dry red chilies
- 1/2 a teaspoon of mustard seeds
- To cook the Dhal curry
- 1 cup Dhal(lentils,parippu)
- 1/2 some water
- A couple of the multitude of different ingredients referenced for treating above(turmeric, curry ;overhang, garlic, onions)
- 1-2 green chillies cut
- 1 teaspoon of Salt
- 1/2 some thick coconut milk

Directions:

1. Treating
2. Cut the large onion and garlic(4 pods)into slender cuts and put away.
3. Add three tablespoons of oil to a container, incorporate the curry leaves, cut garlic, onions, and turmeric powder(1 tsp).
4. Leave it to cook until the onions turn clear over medium heat for 2 minutes.
5. Lessen heat and incorporate the bean stew flakes(1 tsp) or 2 entire dried red chillies, when you see the onions becoming golden brown, add the mustard seeds(1 tsp)and cook for 2 minutes.
6. When every one of the ingredients become golden brown, eliminate the tempered ingredients from the heat and move to a different dish.

7. The most effective method to Cook the dhal curry
8. Wash the lentils altogether.
9. Turn in the washed lentils/daal(1cup) to the container you utilized for tempering(saves washing).
10. Pour in the water(1/2 cup)with a touch of turmeric and a couple of cuts of onions, garlic, green chillies and curry leaves.
11. Over medium heat, let the lentils/daal cook until the water dissipates, this requires 10-15 minutes.
12. At the point when the lentils are cooked, continuously add the coconut milk(1/2cup)and let it stew on low fire. 10-15 minutes, add salt to taste.
13. At long last, add the tempered onions to the curry and blend. on the off chance that you are serving visitors, keep a touch of the treating.
14. When you add the dhal curry to a serving bowl and top the lentils/dal with the leftover temper for a valid, Sri Lankan show.
15. Serve warm with rice and curry.

28. Flaky Apple Tart

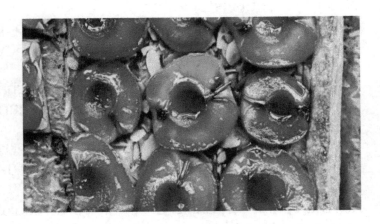

Prep time: 50 min Cook time: 30 min

Ingredients:

- 12 SERVINGS
- ½
- cup cut almonds
- 6
- medium sweet-tart apples (like Pink Lady, Honeycrisp, or Winesap)
- 1
- lemon, split
- ½
- cup unadulterated maple syrup
- ¼
- cup cognac, ideally apple
- 2
- tsp. vanilla concentrate
- Spot of fit salt
- 2
- Tbsp. crude sugar, isolated

- 1
- Tbsp. universally handy flour, in addition to additional for cleaning
- Alternate way Puff Pastry
- 1
- large egg, beaten to mix
- Vanilla frozen yogurt (for serving)

Planning:

1. Spot a rack in center of oven; preheat to 350°. Toast almonds on a rimmed heating sheet, throwing once, until golden brown, 6–8 minutes. Let cool.
2. Lessen oven temperature to 275°. Strip apples; cut down the middle. Using a melon hotshot or teaspoon, scoop out centers.
3. Rub cut sides of lemon all over apples, at that point place apples cut side down in a 13x9" preparing dish. Crush lemon parts over and add maple syrup, cognac, vanilla, and salt.
4. Cover firmly with thwart and prepare until juices are gurgling and apples are delicate yet unblemished (jab through foil with an analyzer or toothpick to check), 60–80 minutes. Uncover and let cool. Increment oven temperature to 400°.
5. In the mean time, throw almonds, 1 Tbsp. crude sugar, and 1 Tbsp. flour in a little bowl; put away.
6. Allow puff baked good to sit at room temperature around 4 minutes to relax marginally. Carry out on a daintily floured sheet of material paper, cleaning with more

flour on a case by case basis to forestall staying and pivoting a few times, to a 16x12" square shape. Slide material paper with cake onto a large rimmed preparing sheet. Trim around sides to fix and clean edges, at that point remove a 1" take from each side (you'll have 4 strips).

7. Brush around edge of square shape with egg, at that point place strips on top, lining up with edges. Trim any shade from corners. Brush edge you just made with egg and sprinkle with staying 1 Tbsp. crude sugar. Dissipate saved almond blend over cake, remaining inside the edge.

8. Delicately organize apples on top of almond combination; save squeezes left in dish. Chill tart 15 minutes.

9. Heat tart 20 minutes. Lessen oven temperature to 350° and keep on heating until baked good is profound golden brown and puffed, 45–55 minutes.

10. Then, scratch held squeezed apple into a little pot and cook over medium heat, whirling dish regularly, until sweet (you ought to have 2–4 Tbsp.), 6–8 minutes. Eliminate coat from heat.

11. Eliminate tart from oven and brush coat over apples. Serve warm or room temperature with scoops of frozen yogurt.

12. Do Ahead: Tart can be prepared 10 hours ahead. Store approximately wrapped at room temperature. Reheat in a 250° oven whenever wanted.

29. Samosas

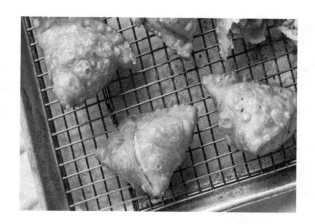

Prep time: 30 min Cook time: 15 min

Ingredients:

- MAKES 16
- FILLING
- 4
- medium reddish brown potatoes (around 9 oz. each)
- 2
- tsp. legitimate salt, in addition to additional
- 1½
- tsp. coriander seeds
- 2
- Tbsp. ground coriander
- 2
- tsp. amchoor
- 1
- tsp. anardana powder
- 3

- Tbsp. impartial oil, (for example, grapeseed or vegetable)
- 1
- tsp. cumin seeds
- SHELLS AND ASSEMBLY
- 6¼
- cups unbiased oil, (for example, grapeseed or vegetable), partitioned
- 1
- tsp. genuine salt
- ½
- tsp. ajwain
- 2
- cups (250 g) universally handy flour, in addition to additional for surface
- Cilantro Chutney and Sweet Tamarind Chutney (for serving; optional)

Planning:

1. FILLING
2. Consolidate potatoes with enough liberally salted water to cover by in any event 1" in a medium pan. Heat to the point of boiling over medium-high heat. Lessen heat to medium-low and stew until potatoes are delicate, around 30 minutes. Channel potatoes and put away until adequately cool to deal with. Strip potatoes, at that point coarsely pound with a potato masher or fork.
3. Pulverize coriander seeds with the lower part of an estimating cup or the side of a gourmet expert's blade until coarsely ground. Move to a little bowl. Add ground coriander, amchoor,

anardana powder, and staying 2 tsp. salt and mix to join.

4. Heat oil in a large skillet over medium. Cook cumin seeds, mixing every now and again, until fragrant, around 1 moment. Add zest blend and keep on cooking, mixing so flavors don't consume, until just heated through, around 30 seconds. Eliminate from heat and add potatoes to skillet, collapsing and crushing into flavor combination to consolidate. Let cool.

5. SHELLS AND ASSEMBLY

6. Mix ¼ cup oil and ⅔ cup water in a little bowl to consolidate. Blend salt, ajwain, and 2 cups flour in a large bowl to join. Mix in 66% of oil-water blend until consolidated, at that point slowly add more, mixing continually, until fused and batter meets up in a ball.

7. Turn out batter onto a delicately floured surface and massage until smooth, around 1 moment. Structure mixture into a ball and firmly wrap. Let rest at room temperature to allow mixture to hydrate, 30 minutes.

8. Using your hands, move mixture on a floured surface to a 16"- long log. Cut transversely into 8 pieces. Fold each piece into a ball, at that point smooth to a circle. Carry out each plate to a 6"- distance across round, tidying regularly with flour. Slice each round down the middle.

9. Working with each crescent in turn and keeping a bowl of water helpful, dunk at the tip of your finger into water and soak straight side of batter. Pull up corners of straight side and cover the edges somewhat to shape a cone,

leaving adjusted side open; push down on the little opening that structures at the lower part of the cone with your finger to seal. Press covering sides of cone together to seal (be intensive; you don't need the samosa to self-destruct while fricasseeing). Load up with potato blend, delicately driving into cone with the rear of a spoon to smaller, until about ½" from the top. Press top edges of cone together to encase filling and seal.

10. Lay samosa on a spotless work surface. Press down on recently fixed edge of cone with the side of your hand, measuring your palm around the filling. Using your other hand, twist samosa upstanding so pointed end is looking up. Move to a heating dish or shallow bowl. Rehash with residual batter and filling. Allow samosas to sit upstanding all alone around 10 minutes (this progression loosens up the gluten and guarantees the samosas will not explode while browning).

11. Empty leftover 6 cups oil into a 4–6-qt. Dutch oven or large hefty pot fitted with a profound fry thermometer. Heat over medium-high until thermometer registers 375°. Working in bunches of 3–5, fry samosas until profound golden brown, around 5 minutes. Using an opened spoon, move samosas to a paper-towel-lined wire rack set inside a preparing sheet and let channel.

12. Move samosas to a platter. Present with tamarind and cilantro chutney close by (if using).

30. Enchiladas Divorciadas

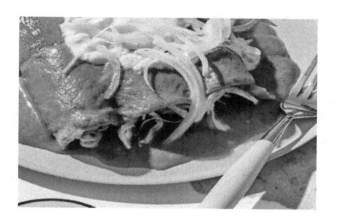

Prep time: 40 min Cook time: 15 min

Ingredients:

- 4 SERVINGS
- SALSA VERDE
- 1
- Tbsp. vegetable oil
- ½
- white onion, coarsely chopped
- 4
- garlic cloves, squashed
- 3
- little serrano chiles, split longwise, seeds eliminated whenever wanted
- 12
- oz. tomatillos (6–7), husks eliminated, washed, split
- 1

- cup cilantro leaves with delicate stems
- Legitimate salt
- SALSA ROJA
- 1
- Tbsp. vegetable oil
- ¼
- white onion, coarsely chopped
- 1
- garlic clove, squashed
- 3
- guajillo chiles, seeds eliminated
- 2
- dried chiles de árbol (optional; exclude for a milder sauce)
- 3
- plum tomatoes, quartered
- Legitimate salt
- ENCHILADA ASSEMBLY
- 1
- 3½–4-lb. chicken
- 6
- narrows leaves
- 1
- tsp. allspice berries
- Legitimate salt
- ½
- cup crème fraîche
- ⅓
- cup disintegrated queso fresco
- ½
- cup vegetable oil
- 12
- 6" corn tortillas
- Cut white onion (for serving)

Arrangement:

1. SALSA VERDE
2. Heat oil in a large pot over medium. Cook onion and garlic, mixing every so often, until beginning to mollify, around 5 minutes. Add chiles and cook, mixing incidentally, until onion is delicately browned and vegetables are delicate, around 5 minutes. Add tomatillos and cook, blending sporadically, just until beginning to relax, around 3 minutes. Add cilantro and 1½ cups water. Heat to the point of boiling, lessen heat, and stew until tomatillos mellow, 20–25 minutes. Allow cool marginally; to transfer to a blender. Purée until smooth; season with salt. Return salsa verde to pot and keep warm until prepared to utilize.
3. SALSA ROJA
4. Heat oil in a large pot over medium. Cook onion and garlic, mixing every so often, until beginning to mellow, around 5 minutes. Add the two chiles, tomatoes, and 1½ cups water. Heat to the point of boiling, lessen heat, and stew until tomatoes and chiles mollify, 20–25 minutes. Allow cool somewhat; to transfer to a blender. Purée until smooth; season with salt. Return salsa roja to pan and keep warm until prepared to utilize.
5. ENCHILADA ASSEMBLY
6. Spot chicken, narrows leaves, and allspice in a little pot and pour in water to cover by 1"; season daintily with salt. Heat to the point of boiling, lessen heat, and stew tenderly until

chicken is almost cooked through (a moment read thermometer embedded into the thickest piece of chicken should enlist 145°–150°), 20–25 minutes from the time water begins stewing. Let chicken cool at any rate 60 minutes (it ought to be simply warm). On the off chance that you have the opportunity, cover and chill as long as 12 hours.

7. Eliminate chicken from stock. Pull meat from bones and shred; dispose of skin and bones. Spot meat in a large pan and pour in barely enough stock to cover. Put away any excess stock for another utilization. Delicately reheat chicken over medium-low; season with salt.

8. Then, blend crème fraîche and queso fresco in a little bowl to consolidate.

9. Heat oil in a little skillet over medium-high until hot however not smoking. Lower every tortilla in oil sufficiently long to mollify however not so long that they self-destruct, 5–10 seconds each. Move to a rimmed preparing sheet fixed with paper towels to deplete.

10. Working each in turn, fill every tortilla with about ⅓ cup shredded chicken and move up firmly. Spot 3 tortillas each, crease side down, into bowls. Spoon ½ cup of each sauce on far edges of enchiladas. Top with a major spoonful of crème fraîche combination and dissipate onion over.

11. Do Ahead: Chicken can be poached and shredded 3 days ahead. Spot in a little bowl and pour in stock to lower; cover and chill.

31. Stuffed Cabbage With Lemony Rice And Sumac

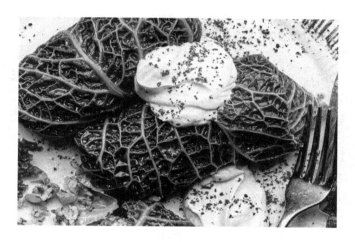

Prep time: 25 min Cook time: 15 min

Ingredients:

- 4 SERVINGS
- 12–14
- large savoy or green cabbage leaves (from 1 large head)
- Legitimate salt
- ¾
- cup long-grain white rice, (for example, basmati or jasmine), flushed
- ¼
- cup extra-virgin olive oil, in addition to additional for showering
- 1
- large onion, finely chopped
- ½

- cup pine nuts
- 1
- cup finely chopped blended delicate spices (like parsley, mint, dill, or potentially tarragon)
- ⅓
- cup chopped golden or brown raisins
- 2
- Tbsp. sumac, in addition to additional for serving
- 1
- Tbsp. new lemon juice
- 1
- large egg, beaten to mix
- Newly ground dark pepper
- 3
- Tbsp. unsalted margarine
- Harsh cream (for serving)
- Fixing INFO
- Sumac, a tart, citrusy zest commonly sold in ground structure, can be found at Middle Eastern business sectors, strength food sources stores, and on the web.

Readiness:

1. Line a heating sheet with a perfect kitchen towel or a couple of layers of paper towels; put away. Working in clusters, cook cabbage leaves in a large pot of bubbling liberally salted water until radiant green and flexible, around 2 minutes for each bunch. Move leaves to a bowl of ice water to cool; hold pot of water for cooking rice. Move cabbage leaves to arranged preparing sheet and let channel.

2. Return water in pot to a bubble and cook rice, blending frequently, until grains swell and ascend to the surface, 3–6 minutes (contingent upon nature of rice). Nibble into a couple of grains to test; they ought to be still somewhat firm (rice will get done with cooking when heated inside the cabbage). Channel rice and flush under chilly running water to prevent it from cooking further. Channel again and move to a large bowl.

3. Crash pot. Pour in ¼ cup oil and set pot over medium heat. Add onion and cook, blending periodically, until mellowed and golden, 7–9 minutes. Add pine nuts and cook, mixing regularly, until nuts smell hot and have marginally obscured in shading and onion is nearly jammy, around 5 minutes. Blend in spices, raisins, and 2 Tbsp. sumac cook, actually blending, until spices have somewhat obscured in shading and are fragrant, around 2 minutes. Eliminate from heat and mix in lemon juice; let cool 5 minutes.

4. Add onion blend and egg to rice and blend well; season liberally with salt and pepper. Crash pot; save. Working with 1 cabbage leaf at a time, cut out the thickest piece of rib by making a slight V-shape; dispose of. Spot 3 loading Tbsp. filling in the middle, running transversely across leaf. Beginning at the base where you cut the V, overlay scored side of leaf over-top filling, at that point overlap in sides and move up leaf like a burrito.

5. Orchestrate cabbage moves, crease side down, in a solitary layer in held pot. Add margarine

and ½ cup water and bring to a stew over medium-high heat. Diminish heat to low, cover pot, and bulldozes until filling is cooked through and leaves are delicate, 18–25 minutes.

6. Gap cabbage moves among plates; shower with oil and sprinkle with sumac and pepper. Present with harsh cream.

32. Vegetarian Enchiladas

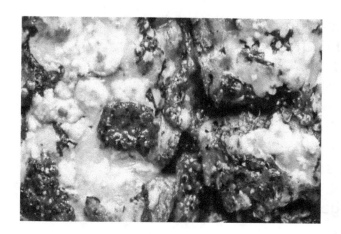

Prep time: 30 min Cook time : 40 min

Ingredients:

- 4–6 SERVINGS
- Singed SALSA VERDE
- 1½
- lb. tomatillos, husks eliminated, washed
- 1
- medium onion, stripped, cut into 8 wedges
- 6–8
- large poblano chiles (about 1½ lb. complete)
- 2
- serrano chiles
- 6
- garlic cloves, unpeeled
- 3
- Tbsp. extra-virgin olive oil, isolated
- 1
- tsp. fit salt, in addition to additional

- 1
- cup cilantro leaves with delicate stems
- ½
- tsp. ground cumin
- FILLING AND ASSEMBLY
- 1
- medium onion
- 2
- Tbsp. also ⅔ cup extra-virgin olive oil
- ½
- tsp. ground cumin
- 2
- garlic cloves, finely chopped
- 1
- pack wavy kale (around 9 oz.), stems eliminated, leaves finely chopped
- Genuine salt
- 1
- 15.5-oz. can pinto beans, depleted, washed
- 4
- oz. coarsely ground Monterey Jack cheddar (around 1 cup), partitioned
- 12
- 5"– 6" corn tortillas
- 2
- oz. coarsely ground Cotija (about ½ cup)
- Cilantro leaves, lime wedges, cut avocado, and hot sauce (for serving)

Readiness:

1. Singed SALSA VERDE
2. Spot a rack in top third of oven; heat grill. Spot tomatillos, onion, poblano chiles, serrano

chiles, and garlic on a foil-lined rimmed heating sheet (it's OK to pack them near one another). Sprinkle with 2 Tbsp. oil, season with salt, and throw to join.

Cook vegetables, pivoting dish and turning chiles partially through, until roasted and rankled all more than, 13–18 minutes. Watch intently, as grills shift fiercely, and generally, in power.

3. Move poblano chiles to a little bowl. Cover with a towel or saran wrap and let sit 5 minutes. Strip off skin with paper towels (don't stress over getting each and every piece). Eliminate stems and seeds, at that point finely hack 3 chiles; put those away for get together.

4. Move remaining vegetables to a blender, eliminating originates from serranos and extracting garlic from skins. Add cilantro, cumin, 1 tsp. salt, ¼ cup water, and staying 1 Tbsp. oil. Mix until a smooth, homogenous sauce structures; you ought to have around 5 cups. (On the off chance that your blender is little, work in clusters.) Season with salt.

5. Do Ahead: Salsa verde can be made 3 days ahead. Move to a hermetically sealed compartment and chill. On the off chance that it thickens, add 1 tsp. water at a time until you have a more slender, pourable consistency.

6. FILLING AND ASSEMBLY

7. Preheat oven to 350°. Finely slash half of onion. Cut the other half into dainty half-moons and put away for serving.

8. Heat 2 Tbsp. oil in a large skillet over medium. Add cumin and cook, blending, until hot and

fragrant, around 30 seconds. Add finely chopped onion and garlic and cook, mixing habitually, until mollified, 3–4 minutes.

9. Add kale, mix to cover in oil, and season with salt. Lessen heat to low and mix in ½ cup water. Cover dish and cook until kale is shriveled and delicate, 8–10 minutes. Uncover and keep on cooking, blending every now and again, until water is vanished, around 1 moment. Add beans and held chopped poblano chiles and cook, blending once in a while, until heated through, 2–3 minutes. Move to a large bowl and let cool marginally. Add ¼ cup salsa verde and ½ cup Monterey Jack cheddar and mix to consolidate. Season with salt; put filling away.

10. Crash skillet. Heat remaining ⅔ cup oil in skillet over medium-high until hot. Working each in turn, fry tortilla, turning once and decreasing heat if oil falters, until puffed and marginally browned, around 10 seconds for every side. Move to a paper towel–lined preparing sheet or plate and rehash with outstanding tortillas.

11. Spread ½ cup salsa verde in a 13x9" preparing dish. Empty some salsa verde into a shallow bowl or pie plate. Working each in turn, dunk tortilla into salsa verde in bowl to cover the two sides. Move to a plate, at that point place a storing ¼ cup filling into the middle. Move up and place crease side down in heating dish. Rehash until you've utilized every one of the 12 tortillas (it's fine to orchestrate them firmly in the container). Pour remaining salsa verde over.

12. Cover container with thwart and heat enchiladas 15 minutes. Uncover dish, sprinkle Cotija and remaining ½ cup Monterey Jack cheddar over, and keep on preparing until cheddar is softened and sauce is gurgling, 12–14 minutes.
13. Serve enchiladas finished off with cilantro and saved cut onion, with lime wedges, avocado, and hot sauce close by.

33. Apple-Walnut Upside-Down Cake

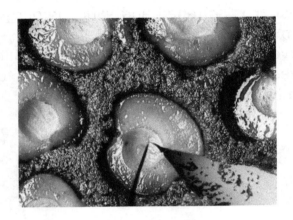

Prep time: 60 min Cook time: 40 min

Ingredients:

- 8 SERVINGS
- 1
- cup crude pecans or walnuts
- 10
- Tbsp. unsalted spread, room temperature, isolated
- 4
- little or 3 large preparing apples (like Pink Lady), stripped, split, cored
- ½
- cup (pressed) light brown sugar, partitioned
- 1
- cup universally handy flour
- 1
- tsp. fit salt

- 1
- tsp. heating pop
- ½
- tsp. heating powder
- ¼
- tsp. newly ground nutmeg
- 1½
- tsp. ground cinnamon, in addition to additional for serving
- ½
- cup granulated sugar
- 2
- large eggs, room temperature
- 1
- tsp. vanilla concentrate
- ½
- cup plain entire milk Greek yogurt, room temperature
- Delicately sweetened, delicately whipped cream (for serving)

Arrangement:

1. Spot a rack in center of oven and preheat to 350°. Spread out pecans on a rimmed preparing sheet and toast, throwing once, until golden brown, 10–12 minutes. Let cool.
2. In the interim, heat a 10" ovenproof skillet, ideally cast iron, over medium. Add 2 Tbsp. spread and whirl to cover; organize apple parts cut sides down in a solitary layer in skillet. Cook apples, undisturbed, pivoting skillet on burner on a case by case basis for browning, until cut sides are golden brown, 5–10 minutes

(the circumstance relies upon the succulence of the apples; juicier apples will take longer). Turn apples over and cook on adjusted sides just until they begin to deliver their juices and the tip of a blade slides through with slight opposition, around 5 minutes. Move apples to a plate, orchestrate cut sides up, and let cool.

3. Add ¼ cup brown sugar and 1 Tbsp. water to skillet and set over medium heat. Mix with a wooden spoon or heatproof elastic spatula until sugar is broken down, at that point cook, twirling skillet sporadically (don't mix now), until thick and rising in a slim layer, around 1 moment. Give caramel cool access skillet.

4. Then, beat toasted pecans, flour, salt, preparing pop, heating powder, nutmeg, and 1½ tsp. cinnamon in a food processor until consolidated and nuts are finely ground. Move pecan combination to a medium bowl.

5. Consolidate granulated sugar, remaining ¼ cup brown sugar, and staying 8 Tbsp. spread in food processor (no compelling reason to wash it) and interaction in long heartbeats until combination is light and smooth. Add eggs and vanilla and interaction in long heartbeats, scratching disadvantages of processor once, until blend is smooth. Add half of pecan blend and heartbeat to join, at that point add yogurt and heartbeat just until fused. Add remaining pecan blend and heartbeat just to consolidate.

6. Mastermind apple parts cut sides down over cooled caramel in skillet, dividing uniformly. Crease batter a couple of times with spatula, scratching sides to ensure everything is very

much blended. Scratch batter over apples and work into spaces around apples. Smooth surface (it's alright if there's just a dainty layer of batter in places; it will ascend in the oven).

7. Heat cake until it is browned across the whole surface and the middle springs back when delicately squeezed, 30–40 minutes. Allow cake to cool in skillet 10 minutes, at that point run a counterbalance spatula or a little blade around the sides of the container to release. Set a wire rack topsy turvy on skillet and flip over to deliver cake; cautiously eliminate skillet. In the event that any apples or cake stick to skillet, scratch them off and press back onto the highest point of the cake.

8. Serve cake warm or room temperature. Cut into wedges and top with bits of whipped cream and a tidying of cinnamon.

9. Do Ahead: Cake can be prepared 2 days ahead. Let cool totally. Store firmly wrapped at room temperature.

34. Broccoli Blanched With Sesame Oil

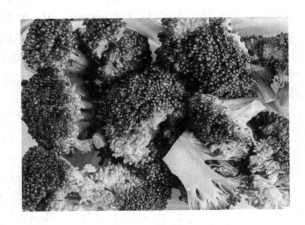

PREP TIME: 10 mins COOK TIME: 3 mins TOTAL TIME: 13 mins SERVINGS: 4

Ingredients:

- ◻1 head broccoli (9 oz, 255 g; florets and stems)
- ◻4 cups water
- ◻1 tsp fit/ocean salt (I use Diamond Crystal; utilize half for table salt)
- ◻1 Tbsp sesame oil (simmered) (or more on the off chance that you like)
- ◻toasted white sesame seeds (for decorate; optional)

Guidelines:

1. Assemble every one of the ingredients.
2. Broccoli Blanched with Sesame Oil Ingredients

3. Separate the stems and florets. Remove the intense skin on the stems.
4. Broccoli Blanched with Sesame Oil 1
5. Heat 4 cups of water to the point of boiling and add salt and stems. Cook for 2 minutes.
6. Broccoli Blanched with Sesame Oil 2
7. When the stems are getting delicate (not delicate yet), add the florets.
8. Broccoli Blanched with Sesame Oil 3
9. Add the sesame oil and keep on cooking until florets are practically delicate, about 2.5 to 3 minutes. Since we won't move the broccoli to frosted water to quit cooking further, we need to take it out before it's totally done. The leftover heat will keep on cooking broccoli.
10. Broccoli Blanched with Sesame Oil 4
11. Channel water. In the event that you like, sprinkle extra sesame oil over the broccoli. Let cool totally and put them in the glass holder for putting away.
12. Broccoli Blanched with Sesame Oil 5
13. To Store and Serve
14. Keep in the fridge for up to 3-4 days or cooler for as long as a month. Fill in for what it's worth or use in different recipes (add to Cream Stew, and so on) I sprinkle sesame seeds when filling in for what it's worth.
15. Tips on How to Blanch Broccoli
16. Do you eat the stems (or stalks) when cooking with broccoli? It appears to be quite essential, yet I need to go over how best to whiten the broccoli and not to squander any piece of the vegetable.

17. Broccoli is perhaps the most regularly eaten vegetables, however numerous individuals actually don't normally eat the stems. Perhaps they look extreme and sinewy? Or on the other hand perhaps they look more enthusiastically to cook with?

18. I learned not to discard broccoli stems when I began to help my mother in the kitchen at a youthful age, and it's interesting how I actually recall it. Under the extreme skin, the stems are not just eatable, they really contain more supplements! Indeed, they are excellent for you. I additionally love that somewhat crunchy fresh surface and I generally purchase the entire head of broccoli. At the point when broccoli is appended with the stems, they keep new more.

19. Since the stems are more earnestly than the broccoli florets, you need to cook the stems first. In the event that you whiten stems and florets together, the florets would be overcooked.

20. The most straightforward route is to add the stems into a pot of bubbling salted water first, let them cook for 2 minutes until they are turning delicate. At that point include the florets and cook for another 2.5 to 3 minutes. You can take them out together once the florets are just about getting delicate. The tone should look new green. Utilize a fork to test the florets for your ideal surface. For most extreme supplements, I prescribe not to overcook.

Conclusion

I would like to thank you for choosing this book. It contains incredibly delicious alkaline diet recipes which can prevent you from chronic disorders as well as can help you in weight reduction.
Prepare and enjoy
Good luck!

CPSIA information can be obtained
at www.ICGtesting.com
Printed in the USA
BVHW091531250621
610374BV00004B/313